Advance praise for

Everything No One Tells You About Parenting a Disabled Child

"I see so much of my own mother in this book and in Coleman's experience. It's the story of a parent who is their child's very first advocate and who is determined to create a more accessible, inclusive, and loving future for their disabled child. Her book contains the necessary tools to begin that future right now."

—Melissa Blake, disability activist and author of *Beautiful People*

"This book should be mandatory reading for all families of children with disabilities, regardless of age or disability type. It positions itself in a way that families should model, a position of listening and learning. What a gift!"

—Rebecca Cokley, US Disability Rights Program Officer, the Ford Foundation (and mom of three)

"When your child receives a diagnosis of disability, most parents feel overwhelmed and confused about how to handle things. In her new book, *Everything No One Tells You About Parenting a Disabled Child,* Kelley Coleman breaks it down, explaining everything you need to know in an accessible way. If you don't yet have a best friend or family member who has traveled this path and can advise you, her counsel will be invaluable."

—Kelly Fradin, MD, Director of Pediatrics at the Atria Institute in New York City and author of *Advanced Parenting*

"*Everything No One Tells You About Parenting a Disabled Child* is the book I wish my mom had when I became disabled at the age of nine. It's a practical guide that highlights the necessity of first-hand disabled expertise, encouraging parents to involve their children in decisions about their own lives, even from an early age. This is wisdom for *all* parents who are raising the next generation of disabled leaders."

—Tiffany Yu, CEO and founder of Diversability and author of *The Anti-Ableist Manifesto* (Hachette Go, 2024)

"I wish this book was around seventeen years ago when our son was diagnosed with epilepsy. We had nowhere to turn and nobody to talk to about it. We caregivers owe Kelley a debt of gratitude."

—Greg Grunberg, actor, founder of TalkAboutIt.org

"When my boys were diagnosed, both times my husband and I were given a stack of papers, a 'good luck,' and a swift quick out the door. We were pretty much on our own. I would have loved a resource like this that could grow with us as my children grew—one that would inform us of all the assistance, materials, programs, and services they could qualify for."

—Tiffany Hammond, autistic advocate, writer/creator of Fidgets and Fries, and author of #1 *New York Times* bestseller *A Day with No Words*

Everything No One Tells You About Parenting a Disabled Child

Everything No One Tells You About Parenting a Disabled Child

Your Guide to the Essential Systems, Services, and Supports

Kelley Coleman

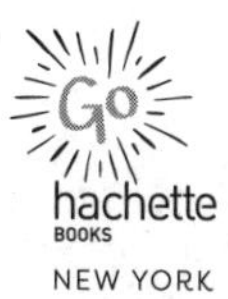

NEW YORK

Cover design by Amanda Kain

Hachette Go, an imprint of Hachette Books
Hachette Book Group
1290 Avenue of the Americas
New York, NY 10104
HachetteGo.com
Facebook.com/HachetteGo
Instagram.com/HachetteGo

First Edition: March 2024

Published by Hachette Go, an imprint of Hachette Book Group, Inc. The Hachette Go name and logo is a trademark of the Hachette Book Group.

Print book interior design by Six Red Marbles

Library of Congress Control Number: 2023951439

ISBN: 9780306831706 (trade paperback original); 9780306831713 (ebook)

Printed in the United States of America

LSC-C

Printing 2, 2024

For Eric, Sean, and Aaron

CONTENTS

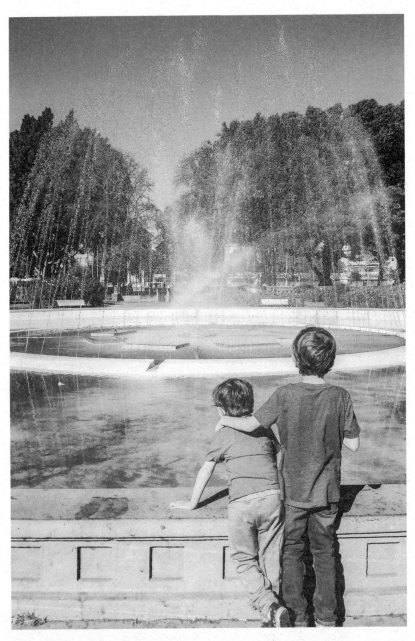

Image description: Two boys standing facing an outdoor fountain, one with his arm around the other's shoulders. A rainbow peeks through the fountain water spray.

Introduction

Welcome. You never thought you'd be here, right? If you're reading this, you're likely the parent of a disabled child, and you're feeling overwhelmed, exhausted, and just plain confused by all the *stuff*. That straightforward path you thought you were on? Yeah, you're on a different path now. The old path doesn't exist anymore. Same here. You're not alone. You love your kid more than anything in the world. But the paperwork? Not so much…

From my own experience parenting two children, one of whom has multiple disabilities, I've learned that no one knows how to do this. When we find ourselves in the middle of it, we reinvent all the wheels. Every. Single. Time. We learn that, in the beginning of this journey, the best place to get real, practical information is often from other parents. And then we become the informed parents. Eventually. This book is your road map to becoming those parents: the ones who figure it out and get it done and celebrate the heck out of your child along the way. Whether you're parenting a newly diagnosed infant or have been the caregiver of your adult child for years, this book is for you.

While I wish I had the magical solutions that would work for everyone, each region, family, child, and disability varies wildly.

There are systems in place. But these systems are often one headache after another. They can feel impossible. If only they had been created by and were run by the people they are serving.

In this book you'll find the things that have worked for me. Many of them will work for you. If what I say doesn't resonate with you, by all means ignore it. Systems, services, and supports are incredibly different from state to state, even under the same federal guidelines. And our children are even more unique. Disability will look different in each of our families. As it should. Every single child develops and grows differently. And your child's path doesn't make them any more or less than anyone else. I have one friend who is presently scheduling college tours for her child, who will be graduating high school with honors. I have another friend who spent the bulk of the past year in a hospital room with her child, who remained hospitalized for months for multiple surgeries and pain management. While both families are experiencing life with a disabled child, those experiences clearly impact life differently, even with amazing parents who love their kids passionately. My friend Jill recently described it by saying, "We are all in the same ocean, but in very different boats." Some days I'm not sure what boat I'll be getting into. They all float. I just have a hard time paddling some of them.

And the paddling looks different for me than it does for you. What do I mean by that? I mean that we all bring our own life experience to our parenting and to how we navigate the waters. Added to that is the very real bias that many families face, not only against people with disabilities, but also bias based on race, education, income, and many more factors. Bias too often impacts the ability to access necessary supports and services. For example, a 2021 report from the California Department of Developmental Services showed that Latino clients receive, on average,

41 cents of Regional Center funding for every dollar spent on white clients. The US Department of Education Office of Special Education and Rehabilitative Services states on their website, "Black or African American students with disabilities are more likely to be identified with intellectual disability or emotional disturbance than all students with disabilities and more likely to receive a disciplinary removal than all students with disabilities." In my conversation with SpEducational executive director and founder Lisa Mosko Barros, she cited her own clients whose disabilities have gone undiagnosed and unaddressed due to evaluators incorrectly assuming learning deficits were due to a child's culture or the language spoken in the child's home rather than a very real disability. Mosko Barros also spoke of the privilege of who can afford independent evaluations, second opinions, extra therapies, lawyers, and to live within the boundaries of a well-resourced school. She acknowledges that families can sometimes figure this out, but that it can be a challenge. "If you don't have the education, you need time," she said. "And time is a privilege." In my own family, I have seen the privilege of time work to my child's advantage. I have been able to take the time to learn, to figure out, and to make things happen so that my child receives the supports he needs. Added to that, I acknowledge that I have other privileges including race, education, income security, and a network of supportive friends and family. And all of this is still really hard for me. It's hard every single day. Is loving my child hard? Nope, never. But all this paperwork? Yeah, it sucks. My aim with this book is to save others much of the time, money, and stress that I wasted learning this stuff. I hope to give others information they can use both to support their children and to confront the bias they will face along the way. We're not all in the same boat. Let's help each other paddle. For the sake of *all* of our kids.

This book isn't about offering one perfect solution. Disability isn't a problem to solve. The problem we need to solve is the lack of sufficient, accessible support. For everyone. This book is not intended as medical or legal advice, as I am neither a doctor nor a lawyer. It's a guide to the basics, so you can ask better questions, get better answers, and find better solutions—with your child as involved as possible in the decisions that will impact their life. Think of this book as a much-needed **You Are Here** on the map of your new life. Where you go from here is up to you.

My child has a rare, undiagnosed genetic syndrome. Odds are our kids are very different—and also have many similarities. Just like all of us parents. As a fellow parent, I don't know what your child needs. But I do know what *you* need: information you can understand and use. I'm not here to help your child. I'm here to help *you*.

Here's how:

The Chapters

Chapters can be read in any order. They are:

- Getting Comfortable with Disability
- Diagnosis
- Working with Your Medical Team
- Therapies
- Insurance and Government Benefits
- Individualized Education Programs (IEPs)
- School
- Disability Rights and Advocacy
- Financial Planning and Future Care Plans
- Inclusion in Your Community
- What This Looks Like for You as a Parent Caregiver

Every chapter includes a personal story and photo, including image descriptions accompanying the photos to increase access for visually impaired readers. Then we dive into:

The Basics

Where to begin, what to ask, and how to get started—this is the foundational information you need to know. The information given is the tip of a gigantic iceberg.

What Worked for Me

I need actionable steps, and I'm sharing mine with you. There are a **lot** of things you can do. Start with one thing. Know that there will always be more to do. And celebrate every single, tiny thing you accomplish. Even if it's just that everyone in your house wore pants today. Bonus points if that includes the dog.

Expert Insight

Remember when I said I'm neither a doctor nor a lawyer? Well, many of the experts featured in this book are. In fact, they're the best at what they do. You will gather your own team of experts, but until then, allow me to share mine with you. Many of the experts here are disabled themselves and/or are the parents or siblings of disabled individuals. The experts featured here speak as individuals, and not on behalf of the organizations with which they are affiliated. Each chapter includes key insights from my conversations with experts, with the full conversations appearing in the Appendix.

Letter to Myself

Turns out you're not the only one feeling *all* the things. In these letters, fellow parents tell their stories through letters they wrote to themselves on the day they learned their child was disabled. There is no right way to feel or to be. There's just walking your unique path and figuring it out as you go.

Templates

Over the years, I've created templates that I've used to make the most of doctor appointments, school visits, and a zillion other things. Save yourself time and energy. Use these templates. And share them with everyone you can. Let's stop reinventing the same wheels.

Ask Yourself

Questions to ask yourself at this point in your journey are included in each chapter. You'll have loads more. Before long, you'll find that you have more answers than questions.

Where Do I Start?

When you're ready to do the things, start here: key points from the chapter, made simple. Super simple. Because we're all exhausted. Consider these your action items.

The more you learn, the more you'll understand that this book is nowhere near exhaustive. Not even close. I'm in the thick of the learning process, and I expect to be for approximately forever. Please reach out to me with your additions, corrections, questions, and thoughts. If I'm wrong, please tell me so we can all learn. We are all in this together, to best support and advocate for our children, and to teach them to best support and advocate for themselves.

Also, language has been a major consideration as I've written this book. As language around disability evolves, the best thing we can do is to follow the lead of those who identify as disabled. As a nondisabled parent of a disabled child, I aim to do right by my child, and by those who experience disability firsthand. The word "disability" felt like too much when I started this journey. I now realize that this was because of my own ignorance. I had grown up with the false belief that the word "disability" was negative. Nope, just a naturally occurring part of humanity. The disability community has embraced this word. It's a word that we all need to see and hear. It's an objective part of the description of who my child is, and perhaps yours too. It's important to acknowledge and fully embrace this identity. As we consider language, it's important to also discuss person-first language (that is: "person with a disability") and identity-first language (that is: "disabled person"). People who identify as disabled make compelling arguments on both sides of the discussion. Based on conversations with and the lived experience of a diverse range of individuals and experts, I have chosen to use both person-first language and identity-first language in this book. My great hope is that the word "disability" evolves to always be used without negative connotation so that individuals may identify as they see fit, and others then follow their lead. The disability community overwhelmingly agrees that we need to get rid of the term "special needs," and other words that tiptoe around the word "disability," as though "disability" was a bad word. It's not. Getting rid of the word "special" can be tricky when it's been institutionalized in areas such as "special education" and "special needs trusts." But, when we're talking about humans, let's listen to actual humans and use the word "disabled." Let's listen and learn and evolve.

I also use gender-neutral language whenever possible and aim to be inclusive of all individuals' identities. I may say "parents" rather than "caregivers," because my personal experience is as the parent of a disabled child; however, my hope is that all caregivers and all types of families will feel equally addressed. Because this book stems from my own lived experience, you'll be hearing a perspective of someone whose child's support needs are medical, physical, cognitive, developmental, behavioral, and sensory. My child's experience, however, is uniquely his own, and there are many conditions with which our family does not have personal experience. Remember when I said that I'm neither a doctor nor a lawyer? Well, I didn't manage to graduate from medical school or law school since you read the last few paragraphs. Note that my personal experience is with the systems in California, but I have drawn from experts across the country in order to provide information that will be relevant to you regardless of your geographic area.

Lastly, you'll hear me talk lots about how to best support my child, about how to foster him on his road to being the best version of himself. My kiddo is on a path that is far from typical—and also far from tragic. If you ask me, "What's wrong with your kid?" I'll reply quite simply: "Nothing." According to the Centers for Disease Control and Prevention (CDC), birth defects impact one in thirty-three babies born in the United States. (I hate the term "defects.") And each of those disabilities presents in unique ways, even within the same diagnosis. It's not easy to be on a unique, and often marginalized, path, but because our son is on that path, we're here to support him exactly as he is. I'm not here to fix him. His disability is part of his genetics, so that would be scientifically impossible. It would be easier to change the world. *That* I think we can do. I'm not out to change my child. I'm out to change the world.

How do I plan on doing that? By telling you everything no one tells you about parenting a disabled child.

Use this book to change *your* world. Use it to save yourself time, money, and stress. To ask better questions. To get better answers. To find a space where you are not alone. And whether your path is easy or hard or somewhere in between, to genuinely celebrate your child exactly as they are.

Thank you for bringing me along on your journey.

Let's do this.

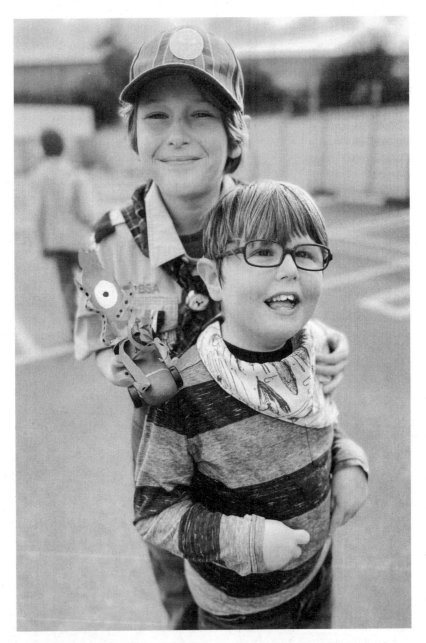

Image description: Two boys stand together smiling. The taller boy wears a Scout uniform and holds a wooden car decorated with a homemade orange squid. The shorter boy has brown hair, blue glasses, and wears a striped shirt and bandana.

CHAPTER ONE

Everything No One Tells You About Getting Comfortable with Disability

Before we jump into all the *things*, there's something we need to talk about: disability. Yes, I know that's why we're here. We're here to navigate the systems and to access the supports and services our children need to live their best lives. We're here to celebrate them exactly as they are. We're here to change the world and climb the mountains and talk about how awesome this all is... right? Well, sure. But we're also here to have real conversations about what this looks like and what this *feels* like. And, I'm not gonna lie, sometimes this feels really hard.

As I wrote this book, over and over again I faced the ableism that I had learned over my lifetime. "What is ableism?" you ask? It's discrimination and prejudice against people with disabilities. It was the "Don't stare! Look the other way! Pretend that kid isn't there!" mentality that led me to feel shocked, afraid, and totally inadequate when I found out my baby was disabled. Those feelings suck. Learning that my child was disabled made me cry every day for months. It upended every bit of my life. And it didn't need to be that way. Before Aaron was born, I would have said I was totally comfortable with disability. After he was born, I learned I was wrong. I had no real experience with disability, and I found myself googling "Blair's cousin on the show *The Facts of Life*." That was literally what I did. Because that was my frame of reference. I was creating fears based on zero real life experience or real knowledge. And that's a terrible idea. No wonder I felt like crap.

Cut to now. That photo of those two smiling kids? Yes, one is holding a Pinewood Derby car that he made to look like a submarine being attacked by a giant squid. And the other one is grinning happily, looking for airplanes in the sky, and living his best life. We all are. (Except for whoever is in that submarine.) I wish I had had this photo a decade ago when Aaron was born. I wish I had known what I know now. I wish I hadn't been taught the false narrative that disability is tragic. I wish I had known disabled kids and adults in real life. I wish I had had the conversations that you'll find in this book. It turns out when you're learning from people with lived experience, disability isn't so scary after all. It just *is*. While no one person can represent the entire experience of disability, we need to have real conversations about ableism, allyship, and inclusion. These are the conversations you need to have to better understand and serve your child. Before we dive into how to navigate all the stuff, let's dive into our own *stuff*. What *stuff* exactly? Everything no one tells you about getting comfortable with disability.

The Basics

What is disability exactly?

The Americans with Disabilities Act (ADA) defines a person with a disability as a person who has a physical or mental impairment that substantially limits one, or more, major life activity. This includes people who have a record of such an impairment, even if they do not currently have a disability. Disability may be congenital (present from birth, caused by inherited or environmental factors) or may be acquired (develops during a person's lifetime). Many congenital disabilities can be classified as "birth defects," though let's be honest, no one likes the term "defects." According to the National Library of Medicine website, "Birth defects are defined as abnormalities of structure, function, or metabolism that are present at birth and result in physical or mental disability or are fatal."

That sounds like a lot of people.

Yep, sure is. According to the Centers for Disease Control and Prevention (CDC), one in four adults is disabled. The exact numbers for childhood disability are tricky to pin down. The US Census Bureau reports that 4.3 percent of children (over three million) have disabilities. Additionally, the CDC reports one in thirty-three children being born with birth defects, as well as one in six children having developmental disabilities. After contacting these organizations and others in an effort to get an answer that reconciles these statistics, I eventually gave up and came up with the statistic that there are *many* kids with disabilities. And that we need to figure out a better reporting system.

That many? But I don't see disabled people when I'm out in the world . . . ?

Disabled people are everywhere. You already know disabled people. You just may not know they're disabled, as their disabilities may not be visible.

Wait, a disability may not be visible?
Correct! Many disabilities are not apparent by looking at someone.

So, that's the opposite of a visible disability?
Exactly. Visible disabilities are apparent by looking at someone.

But I'm not supposed to look at someone because of their disability, right?
You're not supposed to stare like a creepy lurker. You're supposed to acknowledge there's an actual human there, just like you would with anyone else.

Why is my child disabled?
Disability is a naturally occurring part of life and can happen to anyone at any time. There are loads of reasons why disability occurs, from genetics to injury to mysterious science things that I would know better if I was a doctor.

I've seen some TV shows with disabled people, so I know what it's like, right?
Wouldn't that be nice. Disability is increasingly represented in the media, but we all know not to believe what we see on TV. Each individual's experience is unique to them, and the presentation of the same disability can vary from person to person.

I love my child. Period. Is it okay to say that I'm scared what this will mean for them?
Yes. Because your child is in a different demographic than you (unless, of course, you share the same disability with your child). Because there is a ton to learn. Because the future you had envisioned for your child (we all do that) may be different from your

reality. We're not questioning if your child is amazing. They *are* amazing. We're just saying it's okay to feel scared and to acknowledge that this is new territory for most of us. Your child isn't the problem. The problem is ableism and exclusion and systemic barriers at every turn. The problem is all of this *stuff* that you need to learn and to do yesterday in order to access the supports your child needs.

Is it okay to say that I'm afraid what this will mean for me or our family?

Yes, that too. For some families, having a disabled child doesn't change things that much. For others, it changes everything. Some people with disabilities have support needs that require lifetime care, including medical and financial considerations. For most of us starting out, we don't know exactly what it will mean, and we have to adjust to living in the space of not knowing. Part of that is not knowing how your child will be impacted by their own disability.

But I hate not knowing.

Yeah, me too. You'll figure it out. You don't really have a choice. And you love your child. Everything stems from that. Even on the hardest days, that's what will get you through.

What Worked for Me

- Be honest with myself about how I'm feeling.
- Use the word "disabled." Stop using the word "special."
- Seek the expertise of disabled people. Follow disability leaders and organizations on social media, join groups in real life, listen and learn.

Expert Insight: What Do I Need to Know About Getting Comfortable with Disability?

Check out the Appendix for full conversations with the experts featured here.

Rebecca Cokley

Rebecca Cokley is a disability justice activist, currently serving as the first US disability rights program officer for the Ford Foundation. She previously served as the founding director of the Disability Justice Initiative at the Center for American Progress.

- The most important thing you can do for your kids is to have real-life disabled friends.
- We need to use the word "disability." You won't find the word "special" in legislation.
- No amount of education, no job, no country club membership, no anything will protect your child from ableism.
- Teach your child that equal access is not extra and accommodations are not extra.

Oliver James

Oliver James is a motivational speaker, influencer, and literacy advocate who rose to fame when he used social media to chronicle his journey of becoming literate as an adult.

- Your children belong everywhere.
- Connect to your child by being part of *their* world.

Emily Ladau

Emily Ladau is a disability rights activist, writer, storyteller, digital communications consultant, and author of the book *Demystifying Disability*.

- Disabled people need to be leading the disability movement, activism, and conversation. The best thing to do is to advocate alongside us and with us rather than speaking for us or over us.
- Being an ally to the disability community is a journey, not a destination. It's about action—the continued, meaningful action that you take.
- Start from knowing that your child doesn't need saving, your child needs empowering.

Letter to Myself: Christine "Chris" Tippett

Dear 2014 Chris,

You just received Cooper's diagnosis: Mucopolysaccharidosis type I (MPS). There is no cure. Describing this disease, the internet uses terrifying terms like "shortened lifespan," "skeletal abnormalities," and "malformations."

Your world is falling apart. And it will feel like that for a **long** *time. It's okay to be sad and mad. Confused. Scared. In this journey you'll feel more and deeper than you ever thought possible. Talk to friends that want to listen, who are good listeners. Smile and nod to all the folks giving unsolicited advice, then steer clear of them. Your gut will tell you when you hear something that may help. Talk to a therapist. Keep talking to Brian. He's your rock.*

Please know it's going to be okay. It doesn't look like it now, because you are a linear thinker and you need to see how to get from point A to point B in everything you do, before you do it. You're embarking on a new way of life. You don't know the overall plan—you never did, and you never will. The quicker you come to that realization, the better your heart. Let go a bit. You will still be in charge of a ton of life and decisions, but let go of the overall plan.

Let the plan be flexible. See where life takes Cooper and the family, embrace and adjust to every situation.

You will never again feel the way you did yesterday. You will be on a roller coaster of highs and lows forever. You'll have a paradigm shift and find a new normal.

The news of Cooper's diagnosis is going to change every part of your life. Some friends and family are not going to know how to respond. They don't get it, they never will, and it's okay. Don't take it personally. (You'll learn all about empathy and how that looks different to different people.) But please know that there are new, wonderful, life-changing friends to be made and compassionate people leading organizations that will lift Cooper and the family. Other friends and family will step up in ways you didn't know you needed.

No one has your exact situation, and there are few people in this world who will go through what you are going through. You'll find those people and they will be part of your new world.

You have all the skills to take this head-on. Organization, clear communication, and mama-bear compassion. Please take care of yourself. Fill your bucket—exercise regularly, get your nails done, spend time with your people, and get away occasionally.

Welcome to your journey to a new, stronger you. Go live your truth.

Love,
2024 Chris

Templates

There's not really a template for getting comfortable with disability. Being an ally to the disability community is about sustained learning and action.

The CDC offers this graphic on their website (www.cdc.gov) for disability allyship:

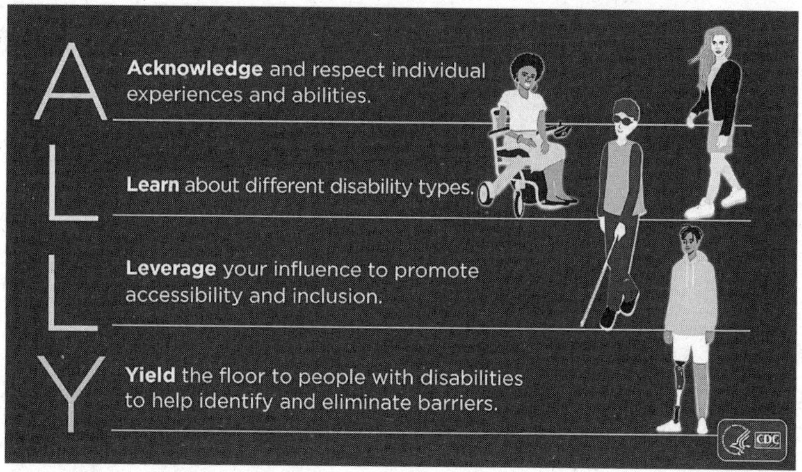

A
Acknowledge and respect individual experiences and abilities.
L
Learn about different disability types.
L
Leverage your influence to promote accessibility and inclusion.
Y
Yield the floor to people with disabilities to help identify and eliminate barriers.
CDC

Ask Yourself

- How do I honestly feel about disability?
- Do I have any real-life friends, coworkers, or role models who are disabled *and* will others feel safe to reveal their disabilities to me (when and how appropriate for them)?
- Do I have friends with disabled children?
- What support do I have from friends, family, and/or professionals? What support do I need in order to best serve my child?
- What steps can I take to ensure that my child is comfortable with their own disability?

Where Do I Start?

- Know you are not alone: and neither is your child. Over three million American children are disabled.
- Be an ally to the disability community—and know that it's about *sustained action.*
- Use the word "disability." It's a word in law, and the word chosen by the disability community.
- Seek the expertise of disabled people to learn about disability.

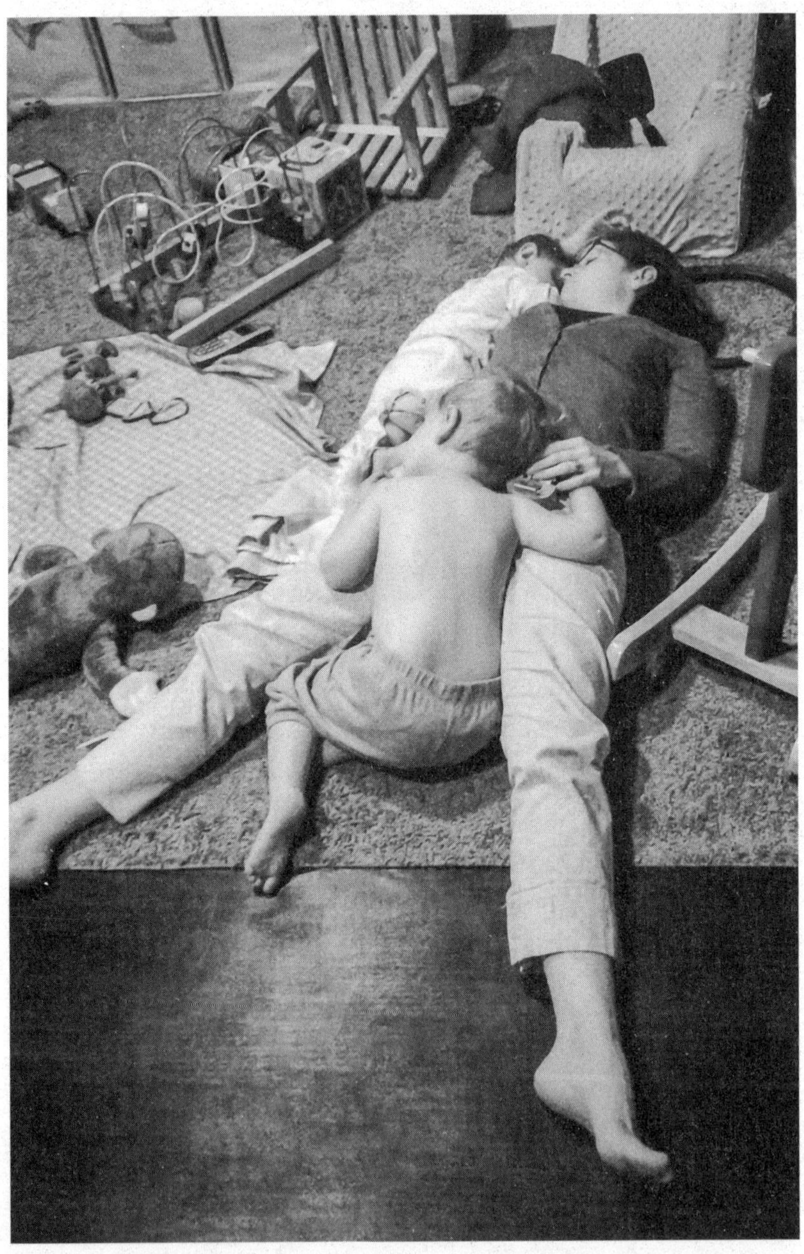

Image description: An exhausted mom sleeps on the floor surrounded by a mess of toys, her baby and toddler draped on her, also fast asleep.

CHAPTER TWO

Everything No One Tells You About Diagnosis

Remember when you had all those plans?

Sigh.

Those were really nice plans, weren't they? Yeah, I had those plans too. They were clear and straightforward and didn't really involve anything much more challenging than skinned knees and convincing my children of the wonders of things like broccoli, flossing, and playing the cello. They were really good plans.

Except that they weren't real plans. Because that's not at all what happened. Sure, we have some skinned knees. One of my children loves broccoli and playing the cello. We're still working on flossing. The other gets 100 percent of his calories via a feeding tube in his stomach and is working on the coordination to hold a toothbrush. I think it's best to keep him a safe distance from the cello. Those things are expensive. Or so I hear. Because, let's be honest, I really don't have time to price cellos these days.

When our son Sean was born, I had the distinct feeling of "I've got this!" and "I'm such an amazing mom!" We stocked up on wooden toys, organic vegetables, and dreams of him supporting my husband, Eric, and me well into our old age. When our son Aaron was born, my gut told me that something was going on with him. I told the nurses at the hospital that he wouldn't eat, that he slept too much, and that something was *wrong*. Every single one of them brushed me off with a smile and an offer of a pink plastic pitcher full of ice chips. I hate ice chips. I'd watch them melt into water while trying to figure out why the nurses wouldn't listen to me. I had the distinct feelings of "What is going on?" and "I have no idea what to do!"

When we brought Aaron home, those feelings persisted. We took him to his pediatrician a lot. Our pediatrician said one of the most important things anyone has said to me on this journey: "Bring your child in here every day if you need to. We will always see you. We will always listen to you. We will always take you seriously." Several months later, Aaron was hospitalized for not eating, and we soon found ourselves stocking up on therapy sessions, feeding tube supplies, and fears of how my husband and I would support this little boy well into *our* old age. All of this while juggling the daily needs of a newborn and a toddler. We were living in a world that suddenly seemed to be spinning much too fast.

This chapter is about diagnosis. Which is ironic, because Aaron doesn't yet have an overall diagnosis. Our medical team agrees that there's a genetic syndrome at play. We've done every appropriate test out there, including full genome sequencing via the amazing Undiagnosed Diseases Network (UDN), and still nada. Within our son's mystery syndrome, he has supporting diagnoses, including autism, cerebral palsy, epilepsy, microcephaly, cortical vision impairment, gross motor and fine motor impairments, intellectual disability, developmental disability, global delays, and sensory processing challenges. Plus he has a feeding tube, a history of chronic vomiting, communication challenges (he's mostly nonspeaking), and is excessively handsome. True story. I write "excessively handsome" on all the paperwork for school and doctors' offices to see if they're reading through everything. It's nice to give them something to talk about besides all the other stuff.

When we started on our path of parenting a child with multiple disabilities, we felt like we were falling into a bottomless pit. There was so much to do and to learn, and I felt totally inadequate. I felt like I was failing my child from day one. I felt alone. I needed someone who would tell me *everything*. I needed someone to sit me down and say, "Here's everything no one tells you about parenting a disabled child." Hey, that has a nice ring to it...

So I'm telling you the thing I needed to hear: You will have to learn all of this. But you don't have to learn it all alone. You aren't failing. You aren't inadequate. There is a bottom to your bottomless pit. And you'll probably hit it at some point. I've been there several times. It's a lot to process, starting with everything no one tells you about diagnosis.

The Basics

Who can diagnose my child?

A good place to start is your pediatrician. They will do standard developmental screenings. Some disabilities are visible and immediately apparent. Some may not become apparent for years. Not all kids follow the textbooks in their development, even typical kids. One of our children didn't walk until seventeen months old but started talking at ten months old. So, go figure. We were jumping with joy when our other son started walking at three and a half years old, and at ten years old first communicated, "No hug Mom" on his communication device.

My pediatrician says my child is fine. I disagree. Now what?

Nothing wrong with getting a second opinion. You're never going to look back and say, "Gee, I turned over too many stones trying to do right by my child." You can meet with friends' pediatricians. You can go to a hospital-based pediatrician. They have a decent chance of taking insurance. You'll probably want to avoid spending too much time on the internet. Because it's the internet. Get the professional opinions you need in order to feel like you're doing the right thing for your child. Maybe there is value to a "wait and see" approach. The answer might be **take action now!** Or the answer might be that you're wrong. It's okay to be wrong.

But my aunt Sally says that...

Is Aunt Sally a neurologist? No, probably not. **You** get to decide whose opinions are helpful or not. Because you're the parent. If listening to Aunt Sally makes you want to whack your head against a brick wall, then stop listening to Aunt Sally.

I've heard of a developmental pediatrician. What is that? Do I need one?

Developmental pediatricians specialize in evaluating and caring for kids with developmental and behavioral challenges. They serve a broad range of kids and disabilities. Do you need one? Maybe. Maybe not. Oftentimes, your pediatrician will be able to steer the ship for you. But, if you feel like you need more specialized care, it could be worthwhile to book an appointment with a developmental pediatrician. If you're looking for one in your area, try:

ASK: Your pediatrician. Your friends. And ask them to ask their friends. Chances are someone knows someone.

CALL: Your local children's hospital. Ask if they have a developmental pediatrician on staff. Make an appointment, even if it's months away.

SEARCH ONLINE: Developmental pediatrician plus your city name. Read reviews.

CONTACT: Your insurance company. Don't be surprised if they don't have an in-network developmental pediatrician. But if they do, tell everyone you know. Including me. Because we're friends now.

So, do I need a diagnosis? I don't want to put a label on my kid.
Lots of folks have lots of opinions on this one. But they're not writing this book, so here's mine: It can be emotional to have someone put a name to the thing that's going on. But it can also open up doors to therapies, services, allies, and insurance coverage. It can also empower a child to put a name to this part of their identity—and to find others that share that identity. If you are able to get a diagnosis, use that information to best serve your child, to connect you with a community of folks with a similar life experience, and to learn how to be the best parent to your child. If you aren't able to get a diagnosis (I'm right there with you), do your best not to lose sleep over it. Maybe the diagnosis will come. Maybe it won't. Allow your child to be your best teacher. You will find your community. You will do right by your child, even if science is still catching up to your unique kiddo.

I just got a diagnosis for my child. I'm a wreck. And I feel guilty about how I'm feeling. Is this normal?
This is a tough one that most of us go through. I spoke about this with Lauren Clark, PhD, RN, FAAN, Professor and Shapiro Family Endowed Chair in Developmental Disability Studies at the UCLA School of Nursing. She had this to say: "It is a momentous change in your expected life journey. This moment stands apart as a defining moment of your life. Any reaction to the news is within the realm of normal. Your child's disability could change many things, or everything, about your future. Parents feel ashamed

that they're sad, they feel embarrassed for their feelings, they feel underequipped, inadequate, angry, mixed with grief. The sense-making process can take a long time. What makes a difference is parents falling in love with their child, watching their child grow, finding hope. Parents do lose hope. They rescue their hope. They regain hope. It's a process."

What Worked for Me

- Create a log of your observations. **Write down** everything that is concerning or that you have questions about. Include dates. Take videos of any observable concerns.
- Take the log (see previous entry) to all doctor appointments.
- Start a file system. Buy or borrow a label maker. Because label makers are awesome.
- Create a log of doctor appointments. **Take notes** at all doctor appointments. Include dates. In writing. Always put everything in writing.
- Make a list of people who could be helpful. Ask them to bring you dinner, or to babysit, or to help sift through the mountains of paperwork. Don't be afraid to ask for what you need. People want to help.

Expert Insight: What Do I Need to Know About Diagnosis?

Check out the Appendix for full conversations with the experts featured here.

Dr. Brian Skotko

Dr. Brian Skotko is a board-certified medical geneticist, director of the Down Syndrome Program at Massachusetts General Hospital, and associate professor at Harvard Medical School.

- Information should be empowering. A diagnosis can be helpful because it leads to more information.
- What parents ask respectfully of their clinicians is not to start with a values statement: "Unfortunately I have sad news" or "I don't know how to say this" or "I regret to have to say this." Anything that conjures up pity or sadness might not be the emotions that are felt or that resonate with the parents getting the diagnosis.
- Do a little bit of self-reflection and self-discovery: How much information do you need, how much volume of information do you want, and who are your trusted messengers?
- Never let a medical professional try to define or reduce your loved one to a series of symptoms or conditions. It's the parents' role to truly know and love their child.

Dr. Emily Bronec

Dr. Emily Bronec is a pediatrician whose practice focuses on compassionate, evidence-based, neurodivergent-affirming care for all children.

- The most important thing is feeling like you have a partner in the care of your child. You need to feel comfortable asking questions.
- There are many things a doctor won't see in a fifteen-minute visit. Think about what your doctor needs to know in order to have the full picture. If you have a nagging concern, pediatricians really need to listen to that.
- Most pediatricians will follow the American Academy of Pediatrics developmental screening guidelines. If there are concerns, your doctor may ask questions about your child's development at any point.

- Any child, even nondisabled children, can fall outside of the range of the milestones.

Letter to Myself: Ashequka Lacey

Dear Me,

I know you are so excited about today. You finally get to find out the gender of your baby. I know you think it is a girl, but it may not be, or it may. I am writing this letter because I wish that I had known what I know today on August 27, 2018.

The last words I remember hearing are "It's a boy." My heart dropped because I wanted a girl so bad. As my son's father went to make a phone call, the doctor stopped him. I knew something must have been wrong. He pointed at the screen showing us that the baby's femur was small and that meant something was wrong. My heart started to beat very fast as I touched my stomach feeling bad because I cried that he was a boy, and now the thought of knowing something may be wrong didn't sit well.

My doctor immediately made a call to the maternal fetal medicine doctor. That's a day I will never forget. The ultrasound was very intensive; we were there for hours. As I waited for the results to come back I had so many thoughts running through my head. The maternal fetal medicine doctor came in and told us that my son had a lethal form of dwarfism called thanatophoric skeletal dysplasia and may not make it.

I refused to believe that I waited nine years to have a baby and I wouldn't be able to hold him. That is the day that my faith was built. I depended solely on God. The options that the doctor gave me were very slim. He told me I should terminate because his quality of life would be poor. He also said if I chose not to terminate, they would set him up with palliative care and put morphine patches on his cheek and he would pass away. Both of those options were devastating. There had to be something else.

This was a test of my faith and it gave me a strength I didn't know I possessed. I decided to advocate for not only myself but my unborn son. There had to be *something else. And there was.*

I want to tell myself I'm proud of you for fighting and not giving up. Your life changed that day for the better even though it didn't seem like it at the time. You made the right decision. You've grown into a wonderful woman. You write books about your son. You started a company inspired by him. You will succeed together. There is *something else. And it is everything.*

Love,

Ashequka

Template: Sharing the Information of Your Child's Disability

Many parents want to share with family and friends that their child is disabled, but they aren't sure how. Is it okay to share this information via email? Sure is. Or phone calls or in person or however you are most comfortable. Parent Jillian Hollingshead emailed family and friends the message below in advance of their son's birth, so that his arrival would be met with **joy**. Whether you learn of your child's disability prenatally or postnatally, the message that follows can be adapted if you choose to share the information in writing.

As many of you know, we will be adding to our family in August of this year. What not everyone knows is that we are expecting a perfect little boy with forty-seven chromosomes. In other words, our little man has Down syndrome. Yes, this diagnosis was unexpected and

> *naturally elicited a roller coaster of emotions. Through the ups and downs, however, one sentiment has remained constant: Regardless of chromosome count, our son is unconditionally loved and very much wanted. We share this news with you now so that our little man's birth may be met with the joy and celebration that it deserves. We welcome best wishes for his safe and healthy arrival, and look forward to sharing him with you all!*

Template: Sample Logs: Parent Observations, Doctor Visits

PARENT OBSERVATIONS: Taylor Johnson, age four months

Date	Observation
2/20/20	Not making eye contact, not responding to light/dark, eyeballs pulsing/shaking often.
2/21/20	Not interested in eating, must be woken up from naps to eat, takes a really long time to eat.
2/22/20	Cries all the time when awake. Can't stop the crying. Seems to have a hard time pooping.

DOCTOR VISITS: Taylor Johnson, age four months

Date	Doctor/Contact	Notes
2/25/20	Dr. Andre Anderson Pediatrician 555-555-5555 321 Address	Referred to pediatric ophthalmologist Scheduled regular visits for weight checks: current weight is XX lbs. Record all wet and dirty diapers; bring notes to next visit

3/12/20	Dr. Kristin Roberts Pediatric Ophthalmologist 555-555-5555 321 Address	Normal eye structures Cortical vision impairment Nystagmus (that back-and-forth eyeball movement I've been seeing all the time) Follow up in three months

Ask Yourself

- Do I believe that my child has/may have a disability and/or developmental delay?
- What signs have I seen? When did I first notice these signs?
- When did I first mention this to my child's doctor? What was the response?
- What local organizations specialize in and support pediatric disability? Who are local medical experts in my child's disability or suspected disability?
- Who do I trust to talk to about this? Where am I getting *reliable* medical information?
- How can I explain a diagnosis to my child in a way that is both factual and empowering?

Where Do I Start?

- Schedule pediatrician appointment.
- Make notes about your child and any specific concerns and/or questions. Take videos if you can. Bring your notes to the pediatrician appointment.
- Reach out to your circle of support. Let them know they're on duty.
- Sleep as much as you possibly can.

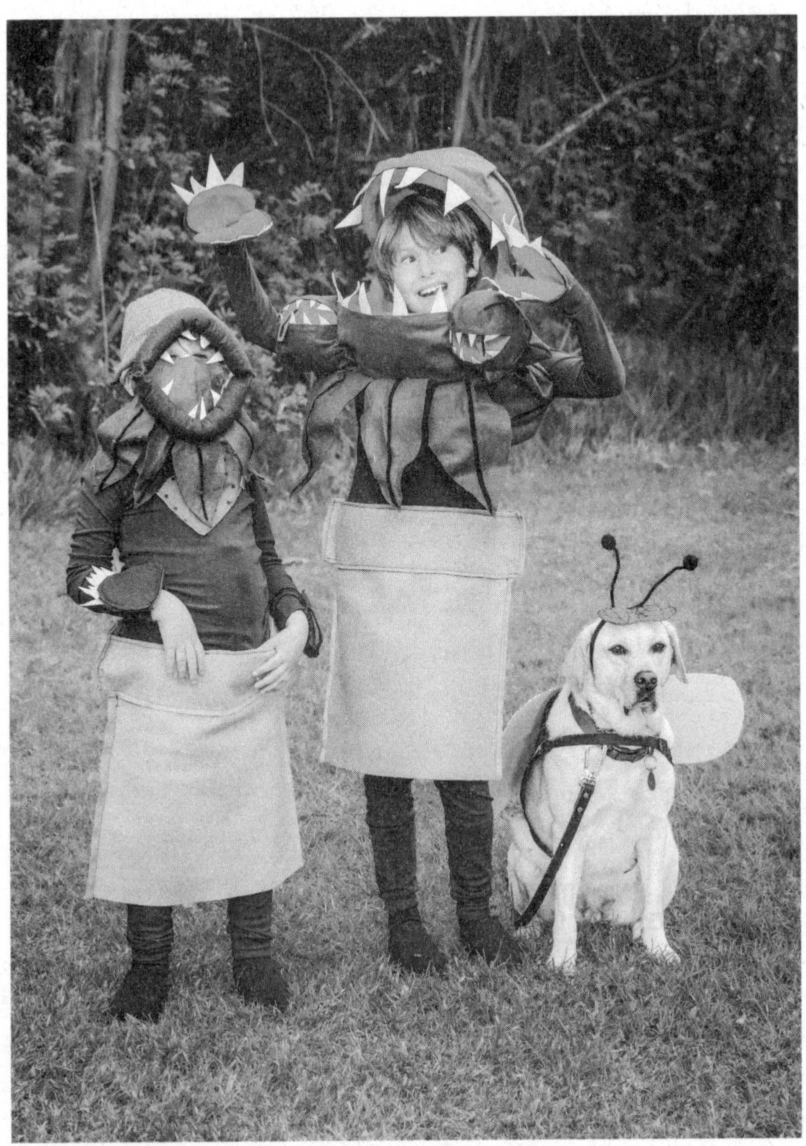

Image description: Homemade Venus flytrap costumes make two boys look like they're being devoured by the plants, while a vaguely annoyed golden Labrador retriever sits next to them wearing a homemade costume of a fly.

CHAPTER THREE

Everything No One Tells You About Working with Your Medical Team

Okay, when I say, "Venus flytrap," what image comes to mind? For me, that would be a sentient carnivorous plant whose main objective in life is to eat live humans, ideally those who kind of deserve it, but really anyone will do. And that's scary. Let's face it, no one wants to be eaten alive by a plant. Clearly, I've seen the movie *Little Shop of Horrors* one too many times. And the play too. So the Venus flytrap in my mind is not only going to eat me, it is also going to sing and to be very, very large. Kind of like my overactive imagination.

My kids inherited many things from me. Strong teeth. Low cholesterol. My inability (or perhaps just disinterest?) to catch a ball. Also my overactive imagination. At no time is this more apparent than during the month of October. We love Halloween. We love it the way some people love the Super Bowl or boy bands or warm Krispy Kreme doughnuts. Every year, the kids get to choose what they will be for Halloween—provided that they help make the costumes. We never really know *how* we're going to make the costumes, but it turns out, with a sewing machine and loads of hot glue, anything is possible. Even Venus flytraps. Their ideas of Venus flytraps are the same as mine, and they were delighted to go to school in costume and pretend to devour their friends. Pretty much everyone has this idea in their head that this is a plant that will eat you alive, and that's scary. But it's fun-scary when it's Halloween.

A lot on our medical journey with Aaron has actually played out like our imaginations about Venus flytraps. I find that I have ideas in my head of what will happen and how scary it will be. I stress out and tiptoe around anxiously, hoping we won't get eaten alive. Because it's all so scary. Feeding tubes? Horrifying. Administering seizure meds? Terrifying. Dentistry for the orally averse? Nightmarish. Well, until we actually experienced those things. Turns out they're not nearly what I make them out to be in my head. Feeding tubes? Totally not a big deal. Administering seizure meds? I can do it while I'm making breakfast. Dentistry? So long as I'm singing "Itsy Bitsy Spider," it's a breeze. I'm learning as I go, but over the years I've gotten better at not creating problems in my head that don't need to be there. I have to remind myself that if I don't have experience with something, I need to learn before I jump to conclusions, no matter what I've seen on some medical show. Overall, things aren't as bad in reality as they are in my head.

Same goes for Venus flytraps. This past fall, I was grocery shopping with my boys and Aaron's service dog. Sean lit up and ran to the floral department. He ran back with an actual, real-life Venus flytrap in hand. Not only was it reasonably priced, but it was surprisingly tiny. Also, it was weirdly adorable—not remotely the bloodthirsty creature I had in my mind. I felt equal parts disappointed and relieved. We named the plant after our checker at the grocery store, Lexi, and it now lives in our kitchen. Every time I look at that plant, I'm reminded that the reality of seemingly scary things is often tiny compared to what's in my head. Nowhere has this been more true than with Aaron's medical journey. Working with our medical team has taught me patience and the value of focusing on what is real rather than jumping to preposterous conclusions (no matter what the internet says). I wish I had known that a decade ago. I wish I had had someone tell me everything no one tells you about working with your medical team.

The Basics

What type of doctor do I need for my child?

There are as many answers for this as there are diagnoses. Speak with your pediatrician about what specialists are necessary for your child's specific situation and for referrals.

So, can I just schedule an appointment with a specialist?

Some specialists will not take new patients without a referral from your pediatrician. Or a referral may help you to avoid a monthslong waitlist. If you're looking for specialists beyond what your pediatrician can recommend, consider sourcing your local children's hospital. Still looking? Call your insurance company and see who they cover—it's always a bonus to get doctors who take your insurance. And anytime you can, ask local friends (yes, those friends on your parent social media groups count).

Monthslong waitlist? Seriously?

It can be a year or more for some specialists. True story. If there's a waitlist of any sort, get on it and hopefully you'll be pleasantly surprised. Ask if there's a cancellation list. Several times, we expected to wait many months to see a specialist, there was a cancellation within a week, and we were in. And be nice to the schedulers. It helps.

They'll take my insurance, right?
Oh, insurance. Sigh. Some doctors will take your insurance, some won't. When you're making an appointment, always ask if they take your insurance, if they are in network, and if not, what exactly are their fees. For some doctors, it will be worth paying out of pocket, others won't be. In general, major hospitals have a decent chance of taking your insurance. But you need to check. You don't want to find yourself with a bill you aren't prepared to pay.

I wrote things down at our appointment, but I can't read what I wrote. Uh…?
Befriend the medical records department! These folks are often overworked and seldom thanked, so your appreciation goes a long way. Find out from your doctor's office the protocol for requesting medical records and if there is a fee. Bring home records and doctor's notes from the appointment if you can. And, yes, take notes, hopefully notes you're able to read later.

Great, so all of these specialists are going to have the answers for my kid, right?
Not necessarily. Every disability presents differently. Some specialists will have solutions, some will monitor your child and will try to head off any major crises. Your specialists will create a treatment plan specific to your child, ideally working together to coordinate care.

But I read about a thing on the internet, so I must know more than my specialist.
Um, no. Also: no. You are the expert on your specific child. Your doctor is the expert in their field. Your combined expertise is what

will make the difference for your child. Ask questions, come prepared to appointments, and *listen*. Too many doctors have told me stories of belligerent parents who fight everything they say. And here's the thing: When you act like that, the doctor still wants to help your child but isn't especially excited to deal with you. If you want a long-lasting, productive relationship with your team (doctors, educators, and everyone else), listen to them—and also listen to yourself. If you wouldn't want to deal with you, then neither will they.

The doctor said to wait and see! I don't want to just wait!
That's a tough one. Sometimes it's the right thing, sometimes it's not. Seek a second opinion if necessary. And know that sometimes the doctor is there to monitor, and that even if you disagree with them, they are doing what they think is best for your child.

While I'm "waiting and seeing," I need help. Lots of it, especially with the boatload of medical protocols that my kiddo requires. What do I do?
Your insurance company or state agency may cover home nursing. Ask about it, and prepare yourself for the realization that there may be a lot of people coming in and out of your house all the time, because you need the support. Home nurses are generally licensed vocational nurses (LVNs). In a clinic or hospital, you may work with LVNs and also registered nurses (RNs).

So, these nurses are magical creatures who will be able to help me do all the things we need?
Pretty much. So be nice to them. Nurses can be a key part of your medical team.

I'm taking my child to the doctor all the time. Do I still need to do routine checkups?

It's easy to forget. But, yes. Lauren Clark, PhD, RN, FAAN, Professor and Shapiro Family Endowed Chair in Developmental Disability Studies at the UCLA School of Nursing, had this to say about preventative care for our kiddos: "As parents, we are often so focused on the acute health problems that preventative care can fall off the radar. Providers need to provide routine care in a way that is tolerable for patients, especially to accommodate people with sensory needs or other disabilities. We can try to keep in mind simple preventative care, simple things like vaccinations, wearing helmets, keeping firearms locked up. Much of healthcare is about prevention and we need to remember that."

What Worked for Me

- Find trusted doctors. It's okay to get a second opinion or to change doctors. The right team is out there.
- Be prepared to change the treatment plan based on how needs are presenting and developing. It's okay to say: "Now that I have more information, my thoughts on this have changed to reflect that."
- Call 911 when you need to. Don't hesitate if your child is in a life-threatening situation.
- Have an emergency bag ready for unexpected trips to the hospital. Include warm socks. Emergency rooms are freezing. Always.

Expert Insight: What Do I Need to Know About Working with My Child's Medical Team?

Check out the Appendix for full conversations with the experts featured here.

Dr. Mark Borchert

Dr. Mark Borchert is a pediatric neuro-ophthalmologist at Children's Hospital Los Angeles, where he serves as the director of the Eye Birth Defects Program and Eye Technology Program in The Vision Center. Dr. Borchert is an associate professor of clinical ophthalmology and neurology at the Keck School of Medicine of the University of Southern California.

- Parents should have expectations that their questions will be honestly answered.
- The best way to deal with your fear is to become educated. You can't let fear prevent you from enabling your child.
- You are not giving up on dreams. You're giving up on preconceptions.

Dr. Gilberto Bultron

Dr. Gilberto Bultron is a pediatric gastroenterologist currently serving as director of Pediatric Gastroenterology for the Los Angeles County Department of Health Services. Dr. Bultron is also the chief of Pediatric Gastroenterology at LAC+USC Medical Center and the director of Pediatric Gastroenterology and Pediatric Subspecialties at Olive View–UCLA Medical Center.

- Too many parents latch on to information that sounds like a cure or that sounds easy, but it may not be based in fact. Talk to your specialist.
- When choosing a specialist, parents should never be afraid of hurting their doctor's ego by seeking a second opinion.
- Let the child see what happens; answer all of their questions. Let them feel like they are part of the process.

Q'Londa Schubel

Q'Londa Schubel is a registered nurse with extensive work experience in home health nursing and hospital nursing.

- Nurses are the bridge between the patient and the doctors.
- Trust your nurse. Communicate. We want you to tell us things.
- Communicate with your child, no matter their age or ability. Be honest with them. Don't tell them it's not going to hurt if you know it's going to hurt.
- When you are dealing with an ongoing issue, write everything down in a log: day, time, symptoms, everything.
- Keep asking questions until you find the information you need. Don't leave without a path forward.

Letter to Myself: Maya Kukes

Dear Maya,

Right now, you may be in shock. You may be hoping there's been a mistake. That any minute the phone will ring and it will be your doctor calling to tell you that the lab mixed up the results. That your baby boy does not in fact have an extra twenty-first chromosome. Even your dad wants you to consider waiting to share the news with extended family. What if your baby is in fact "normal"?

The fact that your father wants you to wait says it all. He's ashamed. But so are you. You've let everyone down. And you did everything right! No sushi, no lunch meat, no raw cheeses. It doesn't make sense. You're only thirty-one years old! Aren't older moms the ones who have babies with Down syndrome? You know it sounds elitist, but you went to a Seven Sisters college and an Ivy League graduate school. What do you know about "cognitive delays"? You have little patience for anything other than excellence and are the last person who should be parenting a child with a disability. And none of the tests picked up anything! There was that one test that said you had a "one-half of one percent chance" of Down syndrome. But you laughed about that. And so did the doctor! But what you didn't realize was that somebody *must be that one-half of one percent.*

It probably won't surprise you to know that many things in the next few months won't go as planned. But since you're a first-time mom with nothing to compare it to, you will blame all the "bad" things on Down syndrome. You'll be bereft that he can't seem to breastfeed, requiring you to pump every two hours, all night long. Sometimes you cry during these pumping sessions because you can't believe this is your life now and this isn't the way it's supposed to be (you will later learn that many "perfect" babies with the "right" number of chromosomes don't breastfeed easily—see: first time mom who blames everything bad on Down syndrome).

But then one day you'll be out to brunch with your five-month-old and he'll start nuzzling at your sweater and you will shrug, "What the heck" and nurse him anyway, and he'll inexplicably latch on as though he's been nursing for his entire little life. This will set off a pattern of him doing everything in his own time, when he's ready, and not on anyone else's schedule. It's an adjustment for your type A, love-of-planning self. But this will make you a better parent, because rather than expecting him to do things at a certain time, you learn to rejoice in just the doing. *When he walks at two. Says his first word at three. Learns to read at six.*

In many ways he will end up being not only your easiest baby but also your easiest child. He will delight in making you laugh. Sure, the toddler years, where he develops a love for bolting (at birthday parties, in parking lots, your very own driveway), will be more than a little stressful, but once he matures a bit, things calm down! And in just a few years you will have another baby, and he will be the kindest, most attentive big brother that you've ever seen.

Although it might seem impossible now, I promise you that someday, having a baby with a disability (who becomes a child with a disability) will just be a part of life. Gradually the grief of what you thought you lost, of what will never be, recedes in the distance. Because the "diagnosis," the "baby with special needs" will become a little boy who builds forts out of couch pillows and insists on wearing a satin cape to the grocery store. Then he'll grow to be a teenager who, when he senses you're overwhelmed, tells you to "choose love, not stress." He will teach you that we are all exactly who we were meant to be.

Love,
Maya

Template: Medical Emergencies

Thanks to fire service paramedic captain Bryan Nassour for this information.

What to do when calling 911 for a medical emergency

- Describe your child's emergency.
- Tell them if your child has a disability.
- Tell them if your child has had an episode like this before.
- Know your child's baseline to compare the current status, including:
  - Medications
  - Diagnosis
  - Cognitive and communication abilities
- Provide a printed emergency form with key information to responders; it should contain:

- Child's name
- Child's birthdate
- Child's social security number
- Parents' contact phone numbers
- Emergency contact
- Pediatrician and any specialists
- Insurance information
- Child's diagnosis and/or medical issues
- Medications
- Allergies, to medications and environmental
- Child's cognitive and communication abilities
- Diagnosis-specific information, for example: full information on your child's ventilator or other essential medical equipment

What to do when you are on the phone with 911 for a medical emergency

- Stay calm.
- Explain the emergency clearly.
- Follow the 911 operator's directions.
- If CPR is necessary, the operator will give you instructions if you are not trained.
- Remain on the phone until the operator tells you to hang up.

Working with emergency responders

- Answer questions and let the responders do their jobs. Give information and be helpful without being overbearing. If you are hysterical or getting in the way of care, they will ask you to step away.
- If the ambulance takes your child to the hospital, you will most likely ride with your child, except in extreme circumstances.

- If you drive separately to the hospital, **do not** follow the ambulance. Your car does not have lights and sirens. You will cause accidents. The ambulance drivers will have to stop to talk to you, and that delays your child's medical care.
- Be respectful of the responders. You might be calling multiple times, and you will develop a rapport, and that will serve your child.

Preparing for medical emergencies

- Have multiple printed copies of your emergency form (at home, car, school, purse, backpack, when traveling, etc.) as well as saved on your computer and/or phone.
- Know your preferred hospital **and** your closest hospital with an emergency room that accepts pediatric patients—not all emergency rooms are certified and legally allowed to accept children.
- Get trained in infant and pediatric CPR. These are different. If there is first aid specific to your child's disability (for example, epilepsy), get trained specifically for your child's needs.
- Have a bag by the door for emergencies, which is packed with enough supplies for twenty-four to forty-eight hours:
  - Medications
  - Diapers
  - Food, especially if your child is on a specialized diet
  - Clothes for you and for your child
  - Cell phone charger

Template: Requesting Information from Your Doctor's Office

What to include: date, patient name, date of birth, medical record number (if there is one with that office), doctor, parent contact information, and information you are requesting.

DATE: 3/20/24
PATIENT NAME: Taylor Johnson
DATE OF BIRTH: 8/8/23
MEDICAL RECORD NUMBER (if you have one): 74356
DOCTOR: Dr. Vargas
PARENT CONTACT INFORMATION: Daphne Johnson/ 333-555-4444
REQUEST/QUESTION:

- I would like to request the doctor's notes from Taylor's last office visit with Dr. Vargas. Please be sure this includes the diagnosis of cerebral palsy, which Dr. Vargas gave us on that visit.
- I would like to request a prescription renewal for Taylor's feeding tube supplies to be sent to our medical supply company SUPPLY INC, fax: 333-555-2222.
- As discussed, I would like a referral for a pediatric neurologist for Taylor.

Thank you!

Templates

Leaving a message for your doctor's office

Yes, I know you've left a zillion messages. But this template is about making it as easy as possible for them to call you back with the information you need. Remember Mad Libs? It's just like that.

> (Beep) Hi, this is (your name), parent of (child's name), birthdate (birthdate, including year). (Child) is a patient of Dr. (doctor name). My number is (your number). I am calling because (your reason). I would like (the outcome you're looking for). If you need to reach me (*or:* Please call me back), my number again is (your number), and this is regarding patient (child's name), birthdate (birthdate, including year). Thank you.

Do you really have to repeat yourself in the message? Yes, you really do. You're making it easy for whomever is writing it down, and you're demonstrating just how great you are at leaving messages. It'll look like this:

> (Beep) Hi, this is Daphne Smith, parent of Taylor Smith, birthdate June 15, 2013. Taylor is a patient of Dr. Johnson. My number is 555-555-5555. I am calling because we're nearly out of seizure medications and I'm kind of freaking out. I would like to ask you to please call in an order for more of his medication XYZ to our pharmacy, Joe's Pharmacy, 555-555-5555. If you need to reach me, my number again is 555-555-5555, and this is regarding patient Taylor Smith, birthdate June 15, 2013. Thank you.

Common pediatric specialists and their area of expertise

- Audiologist: hearing
- Cardiologist: heart
- Dermatologist: skin
- Endocrinologist: hormones
- Gastroenterologist: stomach/bowels/liver
- Geneticist: genes
- Hematology/Oncology: cancer
- Immunologist: allergies
- Neonatologist: premature babies
- Nephrologist: kidneys/bladder
- Neurologist: brain
- Ophthalmologist: eyes
- Orthopedist: bones
- Otolaryngologist: ear, nose, throat (ENT)
- Pulmonologist: lungs

- Radiologist: imaging
- Rheumatologist: joints/muscles

Ask Yourself

- Do I have a pediatrician I trust to be the point person in my child's medical care?
- What specialists do I need now, or might I need in the future for my child?
- How can I contact my doctors after hours or in case of emergency?
- How can I involve my child in their own medical care and teach my child to self-advocate from an early age?

Where Do I Start?

- Assemble your medical team, starting with your pediatrician and necessary specialists. You may need to get on waitlists to see specialists. When you call the office, say, "If you keep a waitlist or cancellation list, I'd like to be placed on that list please."
- Identify your preferred hospital, closest pediatric emergency room, and verify that they take your insurance.
- Create an emergency form. Print multiple copies for home, school, car, backpack, etc., in addition to saving a copy on your computer and/or phone.
- Pack an emergency bag in case of hospital stays.

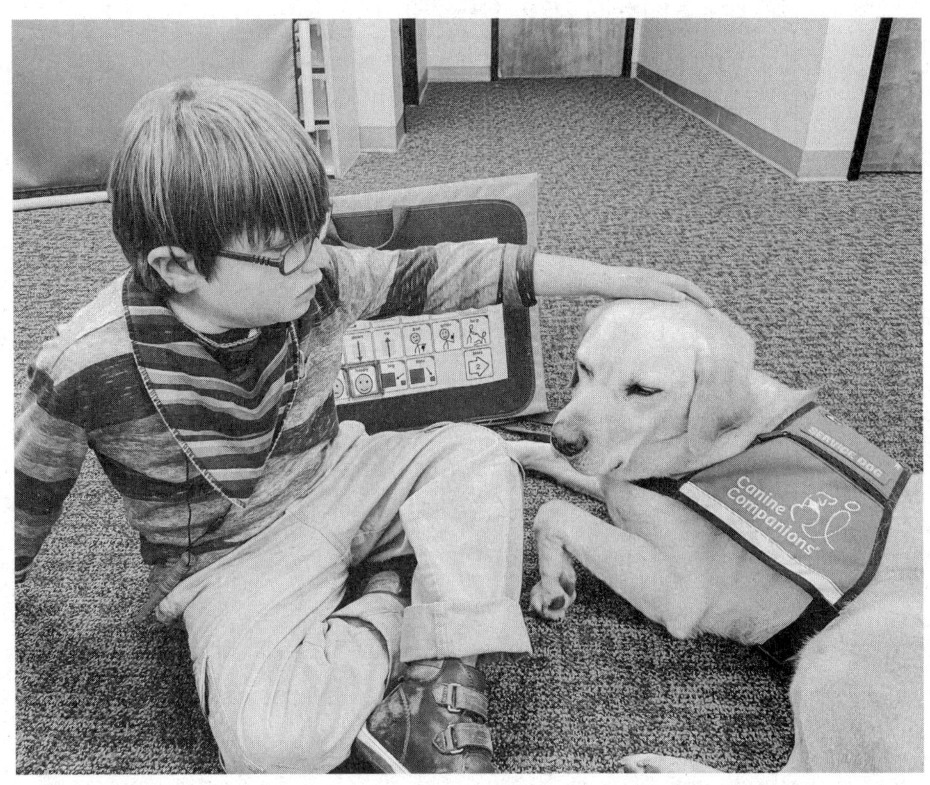

Image description: A boy in a striped shirt and glasses pets his service dog at a therapy center. The dog is a golden Labrador retriever in a blue service vest that says Canine Companions. Behind them is a communication board.

CHAPTER FOUR

Everything No One Tells You About Therapies

As you can see from this picture, everything about therapies for your child will be calm and relaxed and will probably involve an adorable dog and lots of sitting on the floor. Or maybe just lots of sitting on the floor. Prepare yourself for years of sweatpants and ponytails.

Our therapy experience started when Aaron was a baby, and we've been at it for over a decade now. We've worked hard to assemble a team that works well with Aaron, sets realistic goals, and makes the process fun. Some of them even take our insurance. And, yes, it took years to get to this point. We've been on waitlists, we've paid out of pocket, we've driven for hours, and we've tried plenty of therapists who didn't work out. We've learned to be wary of anyone offering us the easy way of doing anything. This is a lot of work. For all of us, but especially for Aaron. We've learned to take our cues from him, since he's clear about whether or not he's happy about doing therapy sessions. The intensive therapy that got him walking? He made annoyed faces during much of it, but he was all smiles every day we showed up at the center. So we stuck with it. The feeding therapy that never worked? He would cry so hard he'd throw up all over the place. Yeah, that didn't last. The whole process has been a huge learning curve, and we're still figuring it all out. Some kids won't need any therapies, and some will need loads. Aaron's therapies have opened up his world by teaching him to access abilities that allow him to participate in life more fully. Walking, yes, but also playing and poking and communicating. Poking is key when you have an older brother. And poking is great when you're learning to use a computer program to communicate and you discover that pressing a certain button will get Mom to sing "Head, Shoulders, Knees, and Toes" every single time.

Through Aaron's therapies, he has also made friends and has been able to interact with other kids, both disabled and nondisabled. They play together in the ways that work best for them. Sometimes that means lying in the grass and giggling at passing airplanes. Sometimes that means listening to the first ten seconds of the *DuckTales* theme song over and over. And sometimes that means sitting like royalty in strollers while going for long walks.

Through the therapy process, I have also made friends with other parents who are driving to the same appointments, using the same feeding tubes, and talking about the same orthopedic shoes (for our kids, not for us, but I'm sure we'll get there soon). I didn't realize how much I needed these connections with other parents until they happened. You need people who get you and who celebrate all the moments along with you: When Aaron first stood for thirty seconds on his own. When he first signed "Dad" at bedtime. When he read an eye chart at nine years old, by pressing buttons on an alphabet toy.

Every single victory is cause for celebration. And that's what we've learned from years of therapies. Celebrate, celebrate, celebrate. We aren't trying to turn Aaron into someone he's not. We're doing what we all do: working hard to become the best version of ourselves. And it turns out that Aaron's best often *is* sitting on the floor, calm and relaxed, with his service dog by his side. We are learning how he learns, and we are seeing him work to be his best self. And, while my best self may not necessarily be wearing sweatpants and a ponytail, I'll go ahead and celebrate that too. Because we're all in this together—along with our friends and our therapists—and that alone is something to celebrate, as is everything no one tells you about therapies.

The Basics

This is all new to me. Therapy? What?

For many parents, this *is* a new thing. Don't fear therapy, be it for yourself or for your child. As with specialists, consult with your doctor as to what is appropriate for your child.

What types of therapies are there?

Many. Loads. More than I can count. Because this book is intended to educate parents on the basics of what is out there, I encourage everyone to look into a variety of therapies to determine what is appropriate for their child. This book does not advocate for or against any particular therapy, because I don't know your child. Though I hear they're very good-looking. Common pediatric therapies include:

- ☐ Language and speech therapy (LAS): Administered by a speech and language pathologist (SLP), this therapy can include help with verbal speech, nonverbal communication, alternative and augmentative communication (AAC, aka communication via a device such as an iPad), and any sort of communication that may be appropriate for your child.
- ☐ Physical therapy (PT): Administered by a physical therapist, PT focuses on gross motor skills. Think big muscle groups

and movements, such as head control, sitting, standing, crawling, walking, running, etc.

- ☐ Occupational therapy (OT): Administered by an occupational therapist, OT addresses daily living skills, including fine motor skills (hand use), sensory support, and others. An OT can have a wide range of skills and specialties, so talk to your OT about what you believe your child needs as well as what specific skills or training they can offer.
- ☐ Feeding therapy: This can be administered by an OT or an SLP specifically trained in feeding. Feeding therapy can focus on the sensory experience, the motor skills necessary to eat, or whatever skills a specific individual may need in order to eat by mouth.
- ☐ Child development: Administered by a child development specialist (CDS), this therapy often looks like play, as it supports a child's development and ability to play and interact with the world around them.
- ☐ DIR Floortime: An intervention generally used with younger children, DIR Floortime is a therapy that works by building a relationship with the child. It consists of an adult following the child's lead by interacting with them on their physical and developmental level. The long-term goal of DIR Floortime is to help the child achieve maximum functionality across all areas.
- ☐ Behavior therapy: Commonly known as ABA (applied behavior analysis), this type of therapy aims to increase behaviors that serve the child's development (for example: communication and play), and to decrease maladaptive behaviors (for example: self-injury and eloping).

In recent years, many autistic individuals have voiced criticism of ABA, based on their own experiences with this therapy. This book does not recommend any one therapy. What is highly recommended, however, is honoring and supporting your child while also taking into account both the lived experience of disabled individuals (in the case of ABA, often that means actual autistics), and what is available to your child, based on your diagnosis, location, and insurance (or other) coverage.

And now tell me about alternative therapies!

There are even more of those. Too many to go into here. Always speak with your doctor before beginning any therapy with your child. Talk to friends, get referrals, and remember that each child has unique needs and will have unique outcomes. If something sounds totally off the wall to you, maybe don't do that. I'm always wary of anything I wouldn't feel comfortable talking about with my child's medical team.

When should my child start therapies?

I'm guessing you know the answer to this one by now: talk to your doctor. You can also have your child evaluated by a therapist to determine readiness and appropriateness.

My child is X years old—I think I started too late!

Don't second-guess yourself. Take it day by day and do your best. You've got this.

So, is my child going to be in therapy forever? How do I know when to be done?

What are the goals that the therapist is working toward with your child? Have ongoing conversations with your therapist about your child's progress. Goals may need to be modified, increased, or thrown out entirely. Don't sweat it. Listen to your child and follow their lead.

Who pays for all of this?

That depends. Some therapies can be covered by government sources (for example: school districts or social service agencies). Talk to your pediatrician about your options, especially for children under age three. They may be eligible for services under a government Early Intervention Program (EIP). When your child enters the school system, some therapies may be included in your child's Individualized Education Program (IEP). Some may be covered by insurance. Some therapists take only private pay clients, so you'll need to break out your checkbook for those (do people even have checkbooks anymore?). Therapy can get really expensive. I know it's a pain to look into all the avenues and options for payment and coverage, but it can save you thousands.

My child hates this therapy. I just want to help them. But they hate it...

Consider why you're doing the therapy. It can be a tough call. Talk to your child if they are averse to a particular therapy—and listen to them. If they aren't able to communicate their feelings, watch their cues, behaviors, and moods when it's therapy time. As often as needed, talk to your therapy team about making changes, accommodations, or even taking a break. Sometimes kids need the time off just to play and be kids, and that's okay too.

This is so much driving around. Therapies, doctors, school...

Yes. Yes, it is. Get some good audiobooks.

What Worked for Me

- Find therapists who have experience with children like mine, will meet my child where he is, and will develop an appropriate plan to meet his goals.

- Clearly communicate my goals to our therapists and determine how progress will be measured.
- Attend my child's therapy sessions and learn from the therapists what I can do to translate the therapy into success and/or knowledge across environments (home, school, in the community). Also, take breaks from attending all the sessions—I need breaks too.
- If my child dislikes a therapy, ask myself why and if it's worth continuing.

Expert Insight: What Do I Need to Know About Therapies?

Check out the Appendix for full conversations with the experts featured here.

Anna Arvisu

Anna Arvisu is an occupational therapist who works with clients with a wide variety of disabilities and support needs.

- Your team should adapt to your child, not the other way around.
- We do not fix children. They're not broken.
- We need to get rid of the "Oh, poor thing" thinking. We shouldn't pity people with different needs or skill sets.

Nikki McRory

Nikki McRory is the founder and executive director of McRory Pediatric Services, Inc.

- Therapy should be a fun process for children. It should feel like play, especially in early intervention.
- Your therapy program should always be individualized. We are all unique human beings, even those with the same diagnosis.
- Parents don't need to be therapists all day with their child.

Bryan LaScala

Bryan LaScala is the chief executive officer of the Neurological and Physical Abilitation (NAPA) Center.

- Let your child show you what they can do.
- Find someone with experience working with children like yours.
- Think about what support you need as a parent in order to trust your therapy team.

Letter to Myself: Elspeth Hetrick

Dear Elspeth,

You have had this nagging sense at the edge of your mind, for a while now, that your sweet, giggly, active baby boy was wired differently, but you were not ready until now to hear the cause: neurodivergence, including autism, sensory processing disorder, and social anxiety.

I don't blame you for being in denial. The portrayal of autistics in the media and medical studies are restricted to a small subset of autistics. Your darling child seems nothing like Rain Man or Gilbert Grape's little brother or Sheldon Cooper or Dr. Temperance Brennan. Besides, our family doctor told you that he couldn't be autistic because he smiles and laughs, makes eye contact, and learned to walk, right on schedule.

It has been easy to write off his behaviors like lining up and sorting toys out by color or size, learning scientific names for different species of frogs at the local pond, and punching his own thighs when frustrated. He was just a five-year-old kid who liked order and precision. Aren't geniuses like that? Maybe he will be the next Einstein.

His anxiety makes sense though. After all, he has spent his entire life struggling to fall asleep/stay asleep, and hassled by acid reflux, and you didn't know those traits were common amongst autistics.

Why don't the standard parenting books tell you that autistic kids often have GERD and may struggle to take naps or to sleep at night?

I want to remind you, right here and now, that these diagnoses have not changed your child. You have the same smart, sweet, goofy kid that you had yesterday.

Now, you are armed with something really important: knowledge. This knowledge is going to help you to advocate for your child's needs, to ensure they have a better experience in school than you did, and to make sure you are not punishing them for things they cannot control.

Stop right there. I know I pushed a button. No, you are not a bad parent. You didn't realize how much this sensory overload was making it hard for him to behave safely and reasonably in public. You thought he could take control and was just choosing not to. You didn't realize **how much** *he needs you to model emotional regulation for him, and to buffer his experiences with his environment, and to plan ahead to ensure he has tools (like headphones, a sensory sack, and a weighted stuffed animal) to help him decompress.*

Those times his aggression left you in tears? They weren't his fault **or** *your fault. His behavior was his way of communicating to you that he had an unmet need.*

Like many autistics, he struggles to identify when he is hungry, tired, sick, thirsty, dizzy, sleepy, hurting, or needs to toilet, and he needs you to help him with interoception skills by recognizing warning signs, and by intervening **before** *things fall apart. In other words, you need to channel your inner Girl Scout and* **be prepared.**

Yeah... I know that is difficult. You already feel like you have to be extra vigilant because he struggles with cooperative play, and gets upset when other kids invade his personal space, and now I am telling you to try to be aware of all his needs, all the time. It sounds impossible. But practice makes perfect, and in a few years you are actually going to be really good at recognizing when he needs to be encouraged to eat or rest or take some quiet time to decompress. It's even going to help you to understand yourself better and to recognize that when you seem cranky, you are really just hangry.

Oh, and... while we are discussing understanding yourself better, let me clear the air. Yes, he is just like you used to be. Yes, he is autistic and anxious and sensory aversive. And yes, you are autistic too.

A lot of the things you are going to do to keep your child safe and happy are going to bother people. Teachers will tell you that you are too accommodating of his need for personal space and that he needs to wait in long lines with his peers. Parents at the playground are going to be annoyed when you let him run around barefoot on gravel (he likes the feeling on his toes) because they want their own kids to keep their shoes on. Your own family members will tell you that you should be forcing him to eat things that make him gag and cry, in order to teach him to be less picky with food.

Ignore them. Do what is best for **your** *child. It doesn't have to be the same thing that is good for* **their** *child. And don't bother trying to win them over. Most of them don't want to understand autism. They want to eliminate it. They only see the difficult parts of autism. They are missing out on all the joys.*

And there are a lot of joys. Your son adores being wrestled with and getting bear hugs. He likes the feeling of being held tightly.

Your boy loves learning new things, and making lists of facts about niche subjects like ancient Egypt and the Titanic. *He adores teaching other people about all the things he learns.*

Your child notices details that others miss. Over the years, he will even help a couple of museums correct inaccuracies or damage to their displays... and he will help locate a LOT of missing pets in surrounding blocks, earning the affection of many of your neighbors. And don't even get me started on his amazing memory for Minecraft *hacks.*

So my message to you is this: Don't grieve or worry or wonder what-if. You have an awesome son. He might be the next Einstein. After all, Einstein was probably autistic too.

Love,
Elspeth

Templates

Preparing to work with a new therapist

Thanks to physical therapist Alyssa Parker VanOver and occupational therapist Kaitlynn Hunker for the following lists.

Questions to ask therapists who may be working with your child

- How long have you been practicing?
- Have you worked with children with my child's diagnosis?
- Have you worked with children with my child's presentation?
- Do you have availability for sessions, or do you have a waitlist?
- How often do you recommend a child comes to you for therapy?
- How long are your sessions?
- Do you take insurance?
- What is your cancellation policy?
- What's the parking situation?
- How will the evaluation/assessment be done for my child?
- Will I get a copy of the evaluation/assessment report?
- How will goals be set for my child?
- How will we track progress toward goals?
- How do you feel about parents observing or joining therapy sessions? Is it required?

- Will you give us "homework" therapy to do at home?
- If my child is struggling during therapy or having a hard time with it, what would you do?
- Are there additional types of therapies that you would recommend for my child?
- Are you willing to talk with my child's school team to coordinate services?
- What is your favorite part about being a therapist?

Sample information for your new therapist

- Child's strengths
- Areas of concern
- Birth history
- Diagnoses
- School or day care the child attends (if any)
- Age of milestones achieved: rolling over, sitting, crawling, walking, speaking, etc.
- How the child participates at home/school/in the community
- Sensory observations:
  - Auditory: how the child responds to sound
  - Visual: how the child responds to visual stimuli
  - Touch: how the child responds to touch
- Your child's motivators
- How your child reacts to new environments or people
- What your family's goals are for your child, and what you hope your child will gain from this therapy

Milestone checklists

Know that your child may not follow typical developmental milestones as defined by the Centers for Disease Control and Prevention (CDC). Nonetheless, you can use the CDC lists as a reference to explain your child's present levels of development and to ask therapists if these are areas where they can work to support your child toward progress.

CDC developmental milestones can be found online at: www.cdc.gov/ncbddd/actearly/milestones/index.html.

Ask Yourself

- Do I understand what therapies could facilitate my child's development?
- What is a realistic therapy schedule for my child and for me, and what therapists are available to work on this schedule? How long are their waitlists?
- Is my child medically able to leave the house for therapies?
- How far am I able/willing to drive/travel to get to my child's doctors/therapists?
- How does my child feel about their therapies? What does my child want to achieve through their therapies, and how do I translate their desires into goals?

Where Do I Start?

- Identify your child's goals and what therapies they need in order to achieve these goals.
- Identify the right therapists for your child. Get on waitlists if necessary.
- Be sure your child has downtime and isn't just shuttling from one therapy to the next. It's tempting to fill their days with therapy. But your child needs time to just be a kid too. And you need time to just be a parent, not just a chauffeur.

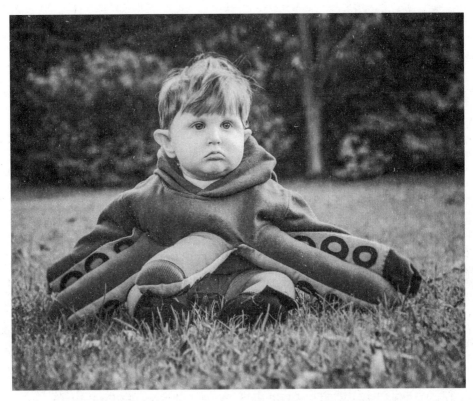

Image description: A male toddler with fabulous wavy hair, squishy cheeks, a serious expression, and wearing a handmade purple octopus costume sits outside in the grass.

CHAPTER FIVE

Everything No One Tells You About Insurance and Government Benefits

Hey, look! A kid dressed up as an octopus!

What does that have to do with insurance and government benefits? Well, nothing. But, by the time most of us get around to slogging our way through the mountains of paperwork to get our kids the care and services they need, we're so burnt out that all we really have the energy for is a photo of an adorable kid with great hair and tentacles.

It can take a long time to even get started pursuing the benefits that are available to you, much less accessing them. For me, it took twenty-one weeks and six days until I actually got my foot in the door, in my case literally.

When Aaron was a newborn, he had his first specialist appointment at two and a half months, his first MRI at three months, and his first hospitalization at three and a half months. Fortunately, all of those were at major hospitals, and we had insurance coverage, so that was relatively straightforward from a paperwork standpoint. It still involved lots of copays and providing our insurance policy member number, which I soon memorized. I bought myself an accordion folder so that I could keep all the paperwork in a neatly organized system. One folder. I thought that would hold years of paperwork. Turns out, it got me through until about Thursday.

By the time we realized that Aaron needed serious interventions to even survive, much less thrive, I had moved from the accordion file to bankers boxes that soon overtook half a closet.

I had meanwhile been trying to get Aaron evaluated to receive state social services. I had been calling and calling, but with no return phone calls. We had been assigned a caseworker (who, I would later discover, knew her stuff but was greatly overworked), but I was getting nowhere. I was having a hard time holding myself together and was routinely failing at simple things like breakfast and wearing socks and remembering the dog's name. I knew that my baby needed help, and that help didn't seem to be coming. So, on a day so rainy that our street was almost entirely flooded, I loaded up my crying baby (Aaron howled in the car for his first year or so of life) and my perplexed toddler into the car, and we showed up unannounced at our social service agency office. Looking back, I don't think that's something people do very often.

The confused receptionist buzzed me up, thinking I had an appointment. And I just showed up in our caseworker's office with two crying children in tow. I was also crying by that point, and we were soaked from the rain. Not my finest hour. While I don't necessarily recommend going this route, it got the job done. Aaron got evaluated the next day, and services started for him soon thereafter.

I had begun to crack the code of what was available for our child. I spent endless hours on the phone with medical offices and our insurance company, and I filled out so many forms that I had to ice my hands with bags of frozen peas.

Nearly a decade later, I still fill out lots of forms, and I've upgraded to bags of frozen vegetable stir-fry when my hands start to hurt. I spend less time just staring at cute photos of my kids (but, come on, that octopus picture is pretty great) and more time doing the work so I can move on to other things. Is it fun? Nope. Ever? Nope. But it can actually be rewarding, especially when you open up the mailbox and find a reimbursement check in the mail. When I was interviewing one of my experts, Leslie Lobel, for this chapter, she said something that I keep thinking about: When she was beginning this journey with her own child, her life felt out of control. The medical journey, the moment-to-moment uncertainty, and the ambiguous future. She realized that she needed something she could control. So, insurance. And, no, we can't Jedi mind trick our insurance companies, though that would be lovely. Leslie cracked the code by learning what was covered and how to work within the system. And *that* gave her control over something, which allowed her to serve her daughter, which made her feel better. It's a thing.

Most of us cower in fear when dealing with insurance and government benefits (raising my own hand here). But we don't have to. I've developed systems and strategies for getting it all done, and I even managed to retain my sanity while changing insurance companies more than once. The maze of paperwork, customer service phone calls, and figuring out all the systems hasn't necessarily gotten easier over the years. I have, however, gotten better at it. Good at it, even. You will too. Once you learn everything no one tells you about insurance and government benefits.

The Basics

Just thinking about insurance and government benefits makes my head spin.

Yep, that's how we all feel. I needed to calm down on this one, so I asked Maria Town, the president and CEO of the American Association of People with Disabilities (AAPD). She had this to say: "It's not straightforward. It requires a lot of research. Parents often don't get access to the best information, even from talking with other families. Often parents get the information too late. Look into state developmental disability councils and the Association of University Centers for Excellence in Developmental Disabilities. It depends on what your child's needs are."

Okay, so the information is out there. I just need to find it?

Yes. It's there. You'll need to figure out private insurance, if that's an option for you (most often through your employer), as well as public benefit options. Oh, and there often can be waitlists for public benefits. And loads of hoops to jump through. You're going to get great at jumping through hoops. We can join the circus together. Judy Mark of Disability Voices United offered that "Children's hospitals have good social workers; they can direct you toward social services in your state." I poked around at our local children's hospital, and it turns out she's right.

Deep breaths. I can do this. Where do I start?

This stresses me out too. So I asked Abbi Coursolle, senior attorney for the National Health Law Program to walk me through this. Her advice on getting started:

- ☐ Government benefits vary greatly, based on what state you live in. There are federal mandates for coverage, but who is eligible and what is covered depends on the state.

- ☐ Call your local public benefits office, local legal aid office, or a social worker who can help you navigate. Talking to a person can often be better than just searching online, especially when you're first learning. These offices can help to inform you about what is available, then you can determine what would benefit your child.
- ☐ With a commercial plan or with Medicaid, you can call and ask for a case manager who can steer you toward the care that your child needs. Having a case manager can save you time, and they can tailor information to your specific situation.
- ☐ Don't feel discouraged when you don't get the answers you need right away. It can be incredibly overwhelming for families. There is so much to figure out. You can't do it all at once. Ask yourself: "What is the priority right now?" Rather than taking it all on, look at all the pieces and prioritize them one at a time.

Can I have both state insurance and private insurance for my child?
Many people do that. If your employer offers insurance, look into that. If your child qualifies for state insurance, look into that. You can choose to have one or both. Get a clear idea of what your employer's health plan covers and what are the coverage limits. Some families have their disabled children fully covered by the state insurance plan (and not the commercial plan that covers the rest of the family), because that state plan may not have limits for medically necessary services that a private plan could have.

How do I even know if a doctor or hospital or therapist will take my insurance?
Ask them. Ideally in advance of your visit. You can also call your insurance company and ask for a list of covered providers for your

particular plan, and if they will pay any amount for out-of-network providers.

What are coverage limits? And out-of-network providers? And all those other things?

If you've been wishing you had more insurance lingo in your life, you've come to the right place. If you have never once wished that, you've also come to the right place. Because it's all important to know. If you're an overachiever (and I'm pretty sure you are), check out HeathCare.gov (www.healthcare.gov) for a more complete glossary of fun-filled insurance terms.

Allowed amount (also known as eligible expense, payment allowance, or negotiated rate): The maximum amount your health plan will pay for a service.

Annual limit: A total dollar amount or number of service visits that your plan will pay per year.

Appeal: A request to your insurance company for them to review and to cover a service that they denied.

CHIP (Children's Health Insurance Program): A program funded jointly by the states and the federal government, CHIP provides eligible children with health insurance who do not qualify for Medicaid or commercial insurance programs.

Claim: A request for payment that your in-network provider sends to your insurance company, or that you send to your insurance company for out-of-network providers.

Commercial insurance: Insurance through a private company, most often by way of your employer. Examples of commercial insurance companies include Anthem, United-Health, and Cigna.

Coordination of benefits: Coordinating which insurance company will pay the claim if you have more than one insurance policy.

Copayment: A fixed amount that you pay for a service visit after your deductible has been met.

CPT code (Current Procedural Technology): A standardized string of numbers (or numbers and letters) that medical providers and insurance companies use to identify medical services and procedures for reporting purposes and claims processing.

Customer service: The number on the back of your card that gets you to people who can answer questions. Or just a number you call to listen to hold music for hours.

Deductible: The amount of money you will pay for services before your commercial insurance plan kicks in and starts paying for things.

Denial letter or letter of noncoverage: A letter from your insurance company stating that the service or equipment you are requesting is not covered by your plan.

Diagnosis code or ICD-10 code (International Classification of Diseases): A series of letters and numbers assigned to a particular diagnosis.

Durable medical equipment (DME): Medically necessary equipment and supplies, such as wheelchairs, oxygen equipment, or incontinence supplies.

Explanation of benefits: The written explanation of what your insurance company paid on a claim and what you must pay.

Full legal name: Yes, I know you know what this is. Be sure that on every bit of insurance paperwork you submit, the full legal name of the patient as well as the full legal name of the policy holder are listed—and be sure those names exactly match the names on file with the insurance company.

HMO (health maintenance organization): A type of insurance plan that pays claims only from doctors contracted with the plan.

Human resources: The people at your job who can help you figure out your insurance plan. Also, they often have the best snacks at their desks.

In network versus out of network: in-network providers are contracted with and accept your insurance plan. Out-of-network providers aren't and don't. You may be able to submit claims to your insurance plan for them to pay out-of-network providers at a set rate.

Letter of medical necessity: A letter from your doctor stating the medical necessity of a certain treatment, piece of equipment, etc.

Lifetime limit: The total amount a plan will pay for benefits over the client's lifetime.

Medicaid: A government insurance program providing free or low-cost healthcare to those who qualify, including people with eligible disabilities.

PPO (preferred provider organization): An insurance plan with more flexibility to use in-network and out-of-network providers without a referral.

Preauthorization: Determination by your plan in advance of a service that the service is medically necessary and most likely covered by the plan (but always make sure).

Prescription (Rx): An authorization from your doctor to cover medications but also things like therapies and medical equipment.

Primary and secondary insurance: Your primary insurance will first be billed. Anything not covered will then be billed to your secondary insurance.

Share of cost: What you will pay after your insurance portion has been paid.

Summary of plan benefits (SPB) or summary of benefits and coverage (SBC): An overview of what the heck your plan covers.

Superbill: The itemized form your healthcare provider gives you that you, in turn, will use to create a claim to submit to your insurance plan for reimbursement.

I can't believe I just read all that.
Yeah, me neither.

What Worked for Me

- Read the insurance policy's summary of plan benefits. And reread it a few more times until it's clear what the plan covers.
- Know which doctors/hospitals/therapists in my area take my insurance.
- Know how much deductibles and copays are, and always confirm that every office has current insurance information on file, including both primary and secondary insurance if applicable.
- Be really nice to the people in the billing departments.
- Know what is available through state agencies—ask my coordinator, and also ask other parents, who will likely be more forthcoming with information.
- Ask parents whose children have needs similar to my child's what specifically they have been able to get covered, both through insurance and through state social service agencies.

Expert Insight: What Do I Need to Know About Insurance and Government Benefits?

Check out the Appendix for full conversations with the experts featured here.

Mary Foley

Mary Foley is the executive director of the Medicaid, Medicare CHIP Services Dental Association (MDSA).

- The eligibility criteria for your state determines if your child qualifies for benefits. The key thing the parent will want to do is to understand: How does the state define disability?
- Prioritize preventative care.
- Have your list of things that you will tackle during the calm times.

Leslie Lobel

Leslie Lobel is the director of Health Plan Advocacy for Undivided, a platform for supporting families raising children with disabilities and developmental delays.

- The way to make it easier on yourself: know what your plan knows from the start. Find out what your plan covers.
- Audit your plan every year: figure out what's going on and if there are any changes from the previous year.
- Always ask the follow-up question: "If this doesn't work out, what would be my next step?"
- Hold yourself accountable. Start a spreadsheet.
- You'll incur short-term stress learning about your plan, but in the long term you'll reduce stress.

Letter to Myself: Effie Parks

Dear Effie,

You're a badass. You know it and you've always known it. Remember who you are.

Your son Ford was just diagnosed with a rare disease, CTNNB1 syndrome. You'll hover over this moment often. You'll get trauma therapy to keep yourself from feeling like you're stuck in a dark and lonely room. You've been gaslit and you've already had to fight for Ford's care and to get to his diagnosis.

This is hard. It will always be hard. You will get better at it—especially if you stay connected, ask for help, and accept all the help that comes your way like you're on an episode of Supermarket Sweep. *Every day you'll have something to learn. Or to unlearn.*

Ford will undoubtedly change everything about your family. People will slow down when they are around him. They will love deeper. His beautiful face will be on a billboard in Times Square. He has a magical power to bring people out of the noise and into his magnetic world of laughter. He's a badass too. And you know where he got that...

Ford will break open a new existence. One that you sure never expected or would invite. Too many days, you're feeling like you're dodging torpedoing lava balls coming at you from every angle. But, even within that, there will be new life-giving joy, hope, and kindness you never thought possible. You will understand the importance of not sweating the small stuff, of creating boundaries, of leaving people who can't get in that hole with you. You will grow.

As you grow, you will help create a community lighthouse that will be a beacon of connection all over the world. You will bring people together to educate others about rare diseases, inspire people to take action, comfort them when they're too lost and isolated or when they're dodging those fiery lava balls. Your work in the rare disease community will bring you to places all over the world. You will stand in front of people and share your story. And the story of your beautiful boy with the most beautiful laughter.

There is so much Joy here. Savor every last drop. You've always known that too.

Love, Effie

Templates

Summary of plan benefits: what you need to know

- When your plan year begins
- Annual deductible
- Out of pocket limits: for family, for each subscriber
- Annual and lifetime coverage limits
- Copay amount
- Coverage for prescription drugs, dental care, vision care, mental health benefits
- If referrals are needed to see a specialist
- Preauthorization requirements
- In-network and out-of-network coverage
- Timeline for you to submit claims to the plan
- Timeline for the plan to process your claims
- Contact information for your plan

Tracking out-of-network claims

Provider	Date of service	Billed amount	Claim number	Money paid to me	Check number	Notes

Calling your insurance company

A helpful guide, brought to you by insurance wizard Leslie Lobel of Undivided.

- Give the representative you're talking to your call back number, right at the beginning of your call. They will call you back if you get disconnected.
- Get a call reference number. This could be known as a call interaction number. Get the representative's name. Often, they will give you their first name and last initial. If you need to call back for the same issue, use your call reference number and if you'd like, you can be reconnected with the person who had previously been helping you.
- Ask for the time frame for resolving the issue. Write down that date and make sure it does get resolved, or follow up (with your call reference number) if that doesn't happen.
- If there is a special authorization you have on file (for services not typically covered), it can be impossible for the next agent on the phone to find it. Ask your representative where exactly it is in their system. Say: "The next time I call, I know that someone else may not be able to find this. Can you tell me what tab this is under, or what system you found this in?"
- Ask: "If this doesn't work out, what would be my next step?"
- Always say thank you, especially if your blood is boiling. If you do lose your temper, own it, and admit you're stressed. Be the reasonable person at the other end of the line rather than the angry, frustrated people they deal with all day.

What to ask your insurance company

Leslie Lobel of Undivided to the rescue, yet again.

- What is the timeline for the plan to process the claims I submit?

- What's the timely filing deadline for out-of-network benefits?
- Is there a preauthorization requirement? How do I get a preauthorization?
- Are there benefit limits? If so, do I get a certain number of visits or service hours?
- Once I hit that number, is it possible to get more? Is it a hard cap, or can I go back to the plan with documentation to request to extend that? Do certain diagnoses allow the number to be exceeded?
- Is the number of service visits combined for occupational therapy, physical therapy, and speech therapy? Or does each service have a certain number of hours allowed per year?

Tracking calls to the insurance company

Claim	Call date	Representative name	Call reference number	Resolution, expected resolution date

Letter of medical necessity: creating a template for your doctor's office to use

Your insurance plan may require a letter of medical necessity in order to prove your child's need (for example, for therapy or for medical equipment). You can help your doctor's office by creating a template.

- Cover letter from you. Keep it brief, explain that the template you are providing is intended to be a helpful guideline for the letter of medical necessity they will be creating for you.

The accompanying template you provide should contain the following fields:

- Child's name
- Child's date of birth
- Insurance plan number, member ID number, group number
- List of points to support the medical necessity of the service
- Medical progress report (your doctor will have this from your child's most recent visit)

What to include in an appeal to your insurance plan

- Progress report from your doctor or therapist
- Prescription from your doctor
- Letter of medical necessity from your doctor
- Cover letter from (and signed by) the plan subscriber to the insurance plan that includes:
    - Insurance ID number
    - Reference number for your denial
    - Concise explanation of your child, their diagnosis, and why this service is medically necessary
    - List of all attached documents

Ask Yourself

- Do I understand the terms and coverage of my insurance policy? Do I have a current copy of my summary of plan benefits?
- Do I know what services (medical, therapeutic, equipment, etc.) are necessary for my child? Do I know where to find coverage information for these services in my insurance plan?
- Do I understand what government resources are available to my child in my state and how to access those resources/benefits?
- Do I understand my state's eligibility criteria for government insurance? Is my child's coverage based solely on disability,

or does family income factor into coverage? Do I need to submit a disability-related waiver through my state social services agency in order for my child to qualify for disability-related benefits?

- If my child is nearing adulthood, how am I preparing them to understand this process, and involving them to the fullest extent possible?

Where Do I Start?

- If you have private insurance:
  - Be sure your child is covered.
  - Find, read, and understand your summary of plan benefits (SPB) or summary of benefits and coverage (SBC).
  - Ask for a case manager or a direct contact (this may not be an option with your insurance, but it is worth a try).
  - Get clarity on specifically which doctors, hospitals, therapists, supports (for example: feeding tube supplies, diapers, etc.) are covered if you do not have this information after reading your SPB or SBC.
- If you have state health insurance:
  - Confirm that your child is covered based on disability rather than based on income (some may qualify under both categories). If your child qualifies based on disability, your state social services agency may need to submit a disability waiver and/or supporting documentation.
  - Confirm if you will be using this state health insurance as your only, primary, or secondary insurance.
  - Get clarity on which doctors, hospitals, therapists, supports (for example: feeding tube supplies, adaptive equipment, diapers, etc.) are covered.

  - If this insurance is your secondary insurance, confirm if you need denial letters or documentation from your primary insurance in order to get services or supports covered.
  - Ask other parents what can be covered via state insurance, because odds are no one else is going to tell you, and each state is different.
- Social services in your state:
  - Identify your state agency providing services to individuals with disabilities. Search online using keywords such as: **your state and disability services** (e.g.: Indiana disability services), or **state name and developmental disabilities** (e.g.: Indiana developmental disabilities) or **state and health and human services** (e.g.: Indiana health and human services). If you can't find the information you're looking for online, call your state governor's office and explain that you are looking for the state government office that serves and supports people with disabilities. Local disability-specific organizations may be able to help you find this information as well. Search online using keyword combinations such as: **autism and your state, rare disease and your state, visual impairment and your state**, etc.
  - Determine if your child qualifies for services. Schedule an evaluation.
  - Talk to other parents about what services are available. Many state agencies will not just give you a list of what is available; however, if you ask about a specific service, they will tell you if that is available. Find out what to ask for by talking to other parents.

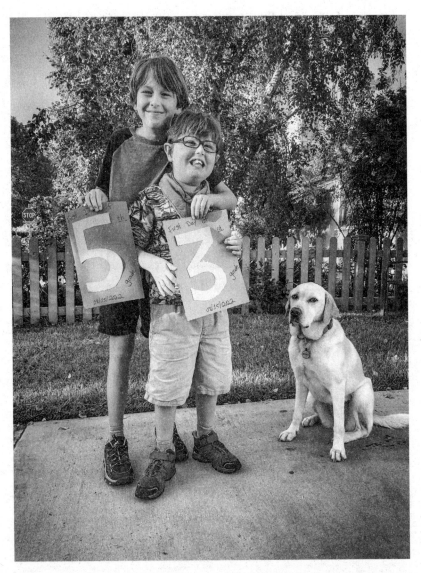

Image description: Two boys smiling and posing outside for their first day of school. The taller boy holds a sign with the number five, for fifth grade. The shorter boy holds a sign with the number three, for third grade. A golden Labrador retriever sits next to them, most likely not going to school.

CHAPTER SIX

Everything No One Tells You About Individualized Education Programs (IEPs)

Our children are presently ten and twelve years old. When our older son attended preschool, he would come home with sand-filled shoes, finger paint on his nose, and chatting about the goats that came to school one day. Actual goats. When it was time for kindergarten, I filled out the paperwork for our local public school, sent him off, and it's been smooth sailing ever since. Because it's just so easy to find the right school for your child.

Unless it's not.

Our younger son, Aaron, is also at a great public school. It's not the public school in our neighborhood, and his preschool years included three schools in three years. The first was an idyllic, inclusive private school. It closed. I cried. I then visited a whole list of public schools, since there were now no private schools that offered the support he needed that were under an hour away. I was tempted to commit to long drives every day. But our son was in the phase of his life we affectionately refer to as "the pukes." It was as bad as it sounds. And, because he was randomly and voluminously throwing up several times each day, an extra two hours in the car wasn't the safest option. His next preschool seemed great. Until it wasn't. The teacher yelled at me for asking which days my son was getting his school therapies and told my husband that I needed to "get with the program." Year three of preschool was at a new public program. Our son's teacher was a remarkable human who would do circle time in English, Spanish, and Armenian to support all of his students. He tuned in to our son to help him succeed, which sometimes meant allowing Aaron to make snow angels on the carpet during lessons. By the end of preschool, I had had about ten IEP meetings. That's *preschool.* I learned **a lot**. And that's where this chapter comes in. Let's save you some of the time I wasted.

Aaron is now in fourth grade, at the same school where he attended the third preschool program, and he's flourishing. It is possible.

It's also important to keep in mind that there probably is no *perfect* school for your child. I spent so much time looking for Unicorn School, only to find that it doesn't exist. What is Unicorn School, you ask? It's rainbowy and glittery and offers things like free tuition, amazing therapists, and expert teachers who dazzle you with their expertise on how to teach your specific child. It's filled with flowers and holiday decorations and is impervious to global pandemics. It's also a figment of my imagination. In my imagination there are actual unicorns there. Or at least a goat or two. After all, my typical child got goats at his preschool (and chickens at his elementary school). So, why should our little guy have to settle for any less? It makes me sad that I couldn't give him Unicorn School. But it makes me happy that we found something even better: a *real* school.

You're going to learn more about the school system than you ever imagined. And I'm going to teach you how to beat the system, right? Well, no. There is no beating the system here. It's a big system. Since you can't beat the system, you need to *learn* the system. You need to play by their rules, because that's really the only way to get your child the supports they need to succeed. For some, that means homeschool, supported by what their district offers.

You will find the best fit available for your child. At a real school. Maybe even one with farm animals. Or not. Because that might not be what your child needs. So, how will you get there? With an Individualized Education Program (IEP). Never heard of an IEP before? Not to worry. You're about to learn everything no one tells you about IEPs.

The Basics

So, what's an IEP?

An IEP is an Individualized Education Program. An IEP is a legal document created together with the parents/guardians and the school that ensures the child receives the necessary supports, services, and placement in order to provide the child with FAPE.

FAPE? What the heck is FAPE?

Welcome to the world of acronyms. You'll have all of these memorized before you know it. And you'll sound supersmart. Let's start with FAPE: Free and Appropriate Public Education:

FREE: You don't pay for it. It's a public benefit for all.

APPROPRIATE: The education is individualized according to your child's needs in a way that allows them to access their education. The word "appropriate" alone could be its own book. You'll use this word **a lot** when you're making a case for your child's education. This is where interpretation happens. Educate yourself so that you are in control of how this word is interpreted for your child. You need to be the expert on what is appropriate for your child. An IEP will often be created and implemented for a disabled child in order to achieve FAPE.

PUBLIC: Public school. If an appropriate public educational setting does not exist for a child, districts may be obligated to pay for a nonpublic (aka private) school.

EDUCATION: School, plus necessary accommodations, including related services (that is: therapies, adaptive physical education, vision services, behavioral supports, medical supports, etc.) that allow the child to access their education.

What do you mean by "access their education"?

According to the Glossary of Education Reform (www.edglossary.org): "The term *access* typically refers to the ways in which educational institutions and policies ensure—or at least strive to ensure—that students have equal and equitable opportunities to take full advantage of their education." For example, if a child is unable to hold a writing utensil, they may not be able to access their education, and so it would be reasonable to request supports and/or services to teach the child to hold writing utensils in order to be able to complete written work. This is where you get to dazzle your school team with your knowledge of your child. Look at what your child will be learning, what is expected, and how your child will be evaluated. Will your child be able to access these things? Is your child able to take full advantage of the curriculum being offered, at the same rate of learning as typical peers? If not, your child will need supports in order to access their education. See how smart you are. You're pretty much a genius by now.

Can anyone get an IEP?

Thanks to the federal Individuals with Disabilities Education Act (IDEA), public schools are legally obligated to provide FAPE for your child. IDEA specifies that children with disabilities are entitled to an IEP if their school performance is adversely impacted by one of the following disabilities: specific learning disability (SLD), other health impairment (OHI), autism spectrum disorder (ASD), emotional disturbance, speech or language impairment, visual impairment, deafness, hearing impairment, deaf-blindness, orthopedic impairment, intellectual disability, traumatic brain injury, multiple disabilities.

My child needs school supports but doesn't qualify for an IEP. Now what?

Federal law to the rescue, yet again. Thanks to Section 504 of the Rehabilitation Act, your child may be eligible for a 504 plan. This plan covers students who need accommodations in order to receive FAPE, and do not qualify for an IEP. If you are considering a 504 plan for your child, be sure to read the IEP information that follows, as many of the same considerations apply.

Cool. So, this is going to be easy, right?

Unlikely. For our son's first IEP meeting, I was given some excellent off-the-record advice from a school psychologist: "Prepare to be horrified." True story. So, if you're ready for that and you aren't horrified in the meeting, then you're already ahead. Don't be afraid. But do be prepared. In many cases, the initial IEP offer is not what your child needs in order to receive FAPE, especially in the case of a child with significant support needs. The school district isn't legally obligated to provide the absolute best thing, just FAPE. So it's your job to know your child, and to ensure that what ends up in the IEP is indeed a Free and Appropriate Public Education. It's not going to be a unicorn. But at least make sure it's a really adorable goat.

How does the IEP process get started?

Talk to your school administrators about requesting an IEP for your child. You should put your request for an IEP in writing and keep a copy of your request for your records.

In order to begin the IEP process, your child must be evaluated to determine if they in fact require an IEP in order to access their education. Children typically enter the school system at age three. If your child was in an Early Intervention Program (EIP) prior to age three, your coordinator should help arrange for your child to transition to school-age services. This will include an initial evaluation.

The initial evaluation for your child could involve many things. For us, it involved me speaking with evaluators in order to give my overview of where my son is in terms of academic readiness, behaviors, medical needs, fine motor skills, gross motor skills, communication skills, vision, hearing, psychological status, and more. As the parent, you should ideally be present for all evaluations. Ask questions. Answer questions to the best of your ability. If something comes out of their evaluation that you disagree with, you can't really discuss it if you weren't there. A major part of the IEP process is that parents are considered an equal part of the IEP team. That's legally part of it. And you should lean on that at every turn. In order for you to be an equal part of the team, you must be allowed to be present for all evaluations and decisions regarding your child. If you are not included, then you are not an equal team member. Your child will be evaluated by school personnel, potentially including district teachers, therapists, psychologists, doctors, and others. The more support needs your child has, the more people will be evaluating your child. Consider in advance how your child does with new people, with groups of people, and if your child would be best served by scheduling the evaluations over multiple sessions rather than one big session. You know your child best, and the goal is to give the district an accurate picture of where your child is right now. Support your child in showing the team their abilities, and if your child is able to do things they are not demonstrating in the evaluation, bring that up with the team. If there are specific concerns you have, or things that you want to be sure are observed during your child's evaluation, write those down in advance, and go down your list in person with the evaluators.

Phew, that's done. That was a lot. Yep. And there's more.

What should I do in advance of my initial IEP meeting?

Tell the district person coordinating your meeting who will attend the meeting from your side. Tell them **in writing**, at least twenty-four hours in advance. Who can attend the meeting? Parents, friends, therapists, advocates, lawyers, your neighbor, your neighbor's plumber. You can invite whomever you want. Because you're the parent and you're an equal part of your child's IEP team. It's your preference, according to what you're most comfortable with, and what you feel will best serve the process of planning your child's IEP. For us, my husband and I always attend. We have brought a friend before, sometimes just for moral support. We also tend to bring one of our son's private therapists, who knows our son well and is excellent in helping the team zero in on necessary goals and supports. When you notify the district who will be attending from your side, also ask for a list of people who will be attending from their side. It will likely be a bunch of people. If you're like most humans, you'll find it intimidating to be sitting across the table from a row of people who have all done this a million times before. That doesn't really make me feel like an equal team member, and that was especially true in the beginning. It actually makes me want to crawl into a hole and hide. Because I have yet to find a sufficiently large hole in any IEP meeting rooms, I like to bring extra people in order to even things out a bit.

If your state allows you to audio record the meeting, tell the district **in writing**, at least twenty-four hours in advance (always in writing, **everything** in writing, ideally as far in advance as possible), that you will be audio recording the meeting. Most likely, you are not allowed to video record the meeting. Bring in whatever device and record all of your IEP meetings—and remember to charge your recording device in advance. It's helpful to have this recording for future reference if you are contesting any part of the district's IEP offer, or if you need clarity on what was discussed. Don't know if your state allows you to record the meeting? Your school may or may not give you an honest answer on this one (it stinks, but it happens). Talking to your local Parent Center for Information and Resources will give you the info you need.

Request **in writing**, well in advance, that copies of all evaluations, goals, paperwork, etc. related to your IEP be sent to you. The district will not send you the actual IEP offer in advance. Because you're supposed to be an equal team member, they can't technically make the offer without you in the room.

They want me to sign things. I should just sign it all, right?

Nope. Remember that. And just in case, here it is again: No. In the IEP meeting, you should sign the attendance form confirming that you were there. There's no reason to sign the IEP document in the room, even if you are pressured to do so. Legally there's no pressure on you. Take the document home and read it carefully before you sign anything. You'll have the option to **agree to all** parts of the IEP, to **agree to some** parts of the IEP, or to **disagree** with the whole darn thing. I always say something in the meetings along the lines of: "Since we will need to take the IEP home to read it after our meeting, we know that we won't be signing the IEP in the room today." That way they don't even ask. Be firm. In our experience, there have been instances when the team in the room has **said** one thing in the meeting but has **written** another thing entirely in the IEP document. So you'll need to read everything. Be sure you fully understand everything, and ask questions before, during, and after the meeting. Feel great about asking those questions. Because you're an equal team member.

These documents are nearly impossible to read. I give up.

Don't give up. They *are* terrible to read. I'm very good at it, and I still find them as confusing as all get out. This is why you should request their reports in advance, and after the meeting take the IEP offer home and read every single page. Maybe yours will be short. Ours is very, very long. When I'm in an IEP meeting, I say this every single time: "Since you guys all know how to read these documents better than I do, I'd like you to please show me exactly where that is written in the IEP document." For every single part of their offer, I ask the team to point to the exact page where that is written and offered. *Every time.* At the end of the meeting, I summarize out loud my understanding of what is being offered, and where to find that in the IEP document. I encourage the team to jump in and correct me when I'm wrong. They do. And I genuinely appreciate it. This keeps all of us on the same page.

That sounds like it takes forever.

Yep. We had one IEP meeting that we broke into two sessions of three hours each. That's not the norm. But it can happen. If everything doesn't get covered in the meeting, you can recess the meeting and schedule a date to reconvene. But **do not** leave the room without a reconvene date scheduled. We made that mistake a grand total of once. Don't do that. Trust me. That said, a reconvene is common and nothing to sweat.

This sounds stressful. Should I bring a lawyer? An advocate? Snacks?

Yes. Maybe. Maybe. Definitely. Our lawyer once told me that if you're at risk of signing the document in the room, bring a lawyer to remind you not to. Instead of bringing our lawyer to our IEP meeting, as soon as the meeting date is set, I schedule a meeting with our lawyer for immediately after the IEP meeting. You might not need a lawyer or an advocate. But you will need snacks. Because who doesn't love snacks. It sets a nice tone. I'm a wake up early and bake some muffins sort of person, so I do just that. Or you could just grab some cookies from the store. Bring napkins if you're an overachiever (I am). It sets a tone of "We're in this together," even if you're just gritting your teeth and waiting for it to be over.

Why does this all sound so awful?

Well, it can be awful. But it doesn't have to be. In a recent IEP meeting, one of our service providers said, "Our IEP meetings feel like a master class in all things Aaron." And he was absolutely right. Meetings can and should be genuinely collaborative, and the parents absolutely can and should be an equal part of the IEP team.

So, how exactly do I make myself an equal part of the IEP team? My mantra: Be reasonable. Be respectful. Be right.

Be reasonable. Know that you are building a plan for your child to receive FAPE. So don't ask for things that are not directly related to your child's education and the supports/services they need in order to access that education. Want to write in there that your kid can bring the family cat to school? Nope, not happening, not reasonable.

Be respectful. Listen. Learn from what the team has observed about your child. Be willing to engage in real dialogue. And be nice. That can be hard sometimes. I get it. Some teams are great. Some, not so much. Can't be nice? At least be civil.

Be right. That's a hard one when you have no idea what you're doing. Most of us don't in the beginning. But you know your child. Be confident enough to ask questions, to get clarification, and to understand what is being discussed and offered. When you ask for services/supports for your child, ask for things that you know they need in order to achieve their IEP goals. You will learn the process and the terms, and this will get easier. Be firm. Do your work in advance. Gather supporting documents if necessary (that is: letters from outside therapists, doctors, etc.). Sometimes the people in the room will have the authority to offer you everything you're asking that your child receive (provided that the team agrees). Sometimes you can all agree, but the team in the room doesn't have the authority to say yes to everything. I have often asked: "If the team were to agree to X, does this team here in the room today have the authority to offer X?" If I don't know the answer to this, then I can't be an equal team member. Ask for clarification on everything. You'll become an expert.

So, what exactly is in the IEP document?

Each IEP will vary greatly depending on the child. That's the individualized part of it. But here's what you should expect:

- **Present Levels of Performance.** Reports from evaluations, assessments, observations, etc. Read through these and see what you think. Maybe the school team is seeing things you're not seeing, or vice versa. If there are errors, be sure those are corrected prior to the meeting or in the meeting.
- **Goals.** These are key. If your child requires services in order to access their education (for example: OT, PT, speech therapy), here's what you need to know: **goals drive services.** The services are only written into an IEP in order to enable your child to achieve the IEP goals. I spend much of our IEP meetings working on goals, both in the room and when I talk with team members in advance of the meeting. Goals are how your child's progress will be measured. Be sure goals are specific. You can also suggest goals to the team. Remember that this is all about school and academics. Keep goals centered on that, or they won't fly. Goals about schoolwork, behaviors at school, safety at school, etc. are all fair game. Goals related to snowboarding or driving a car are not. Some kids have very few goals. Some have many. It depends on the kid.
- **Offer of FAPE.** This is where they offer your kid stuff.
  - Placement: School site location, grade level, and transportation.
  - Curriculum: General education curriculum or alternate curriculum (a non-diploma certificate track that is appropriate for some, but not all, students).
  - Classroom: General education classroom, special education class, or a combination of the two (and the

percentage of time in each room should be specified). If a special education class is offered, it will specify what type, such as intellectual disability (ID), specific learning disability (SLD), autism core (AUT), or others. Ask your assistant principal for a list of special education class options in your district, even the ones that aren't right for your child. Know them all, and you'll be ready in case one of them ever becomes a consideration for your child.

- Related services: Things like school-based therapy, such as occupational therapy (OT), physical therapy (PT), language and speech therapy (LAS), recreational therapy, vision services, adaptive physical education (APE), etc. that your child needs in order to access their education. For any services specified, the total number of hours should be listed (as hours per day or week or month or year), the duration of each session, and if they are push-in (delivered in the classroom setting with other students present) or pull-out (delivered in another room without other students present).
- Additional supports: These vary depending on the child. They could include things like a medical aide for kids needing things such as feeding tube administration or trach maintenance, or a behavioral intervention implementation (BII) aide for those needing behavioral supports, adaptive equipment (such as an accessible toilet seat or changing table), extra time to take tests, adaptive writing utensils, etc.
- Summer school: Confirm if your district offers this, and if it is something you would want for your child. Also confirm that your child will receive the same services and supports during summer school as during the regular school year.

What happens in the IEP meeting?

Expect small talk and signing the attendance sheet. Then the assistant principal will read a long and not particularly interesting document about the IEP process. Humor them. They have to do this for every single meeting, so no matter how boring it is for you, know that it's way worse for them. This is when people will be psyched that you brought snacks. After that, the team will jump in to cover their assessments. They tend to read verbatim what they wrote. And it takes forever. If you've read these in advance, you can participate in the conversation, which makes the experience both more productive and more interesting. You'll also discuss goals and get to ask all your questions. Then comes the last part—the part you're really here for: the offer of FAPE. That's when they offer your kid stuff. Know that it's a discussion with the team, and you are an equal part of that team. Some school teams are reasonable, some not so much. I've been in plenty of rooms where I simply say: "That is unacceptable." Then I eat the fresh muffins that I baked and I stew in silence. Also, if you feel like you need to break down and cry at any point, go for it. It happens all the time. No shame there. These meetings can feel overwhelming. I've absolutely cried during IEP meetings. Though I also cry during Pixar movies, so maybe that's just me.

When everything has been read and discussed and offered, the meeting will end. Be sure that the IEP is closed. That means they've made their full offer and the next step is for you to respond. If the IEP is not closed, do not leave the room until a reconvene meeting has been scheduled. And **do not** leave the room without a copy of the full IEP that includes the full offer. Tell them you'll wait. Even if their printer is on the fritz. They can give you a hard copy and/or email it to you. If they email it, check your email to be sure you've received it and can open the attachment. If your district says they can't email these things, it's all good: Just wait for the hard copy and don't leave without it. And remember not to sign off on it. You'll need to take it home and read it on your own time without a room full of people staring at you. Because that's just weird. Hopefully your home is way less weird.

So I should just talk about all my IEP stuff with everyone, right?
Definitely no. Part of signing your IEP (which is a legal document) is that you are not to share specifics of your IEP with those outside of your IEP team. And remember, social media is not your IEP team.

We'll reach an agreement on everything in this long, long meeting, yes?
Possibly. But we don't. Because of the nature of our son's needs and the red tape obstacle course that is our school district, we have yet for that to happen. And it's exhausting fighting the same fights every single year.

We don't agree with everything. Do I cave in, or do I fight it?
Your call. School districts tend to play chicken to see who will stand up for their kids. If you've done your research to know what is available and what is necessary in order for your child to access their education, you've got a reasonable case. This is the part of the process where I drive around with the windows down and listen to loud punk rock music. The next time you see someone doing that, assume they're a parent in the thick of the IEP process and give them a knowing nod. Our district has multiple options available for resolving an IEP beyond the initial IEP team. The key is to know your child and to know what they genuinely need in order to receive FAPE. Ask your assistant principal or your school district's special education department what your options are for resolving an IEP. For us, that begins with an informal (that is: no lawyers)

dispute resolution process, then escalates to mediation (Lawyers! Time! Money!), and then potentially a hearing (More lawyers! More time! More money!).

Lawyers scare me.

I used to say that too. Then I had an initial consultation with our lawyer, and my mind was totally changed. The right lawyer will listen to you, will learn about your child and their support needs, and will steer you toward what is reasonable and necessary for your child to access their education. Talk to your lawyer in advance about fees, including if you go to mediation or a hearing what the total cost will be to you.

Advocates sound less scary.

Advocates are an option for those who seek extra support but do not require a lawyer. As with lawyers, have an initial consultation to see if you feel comfortable working with this person, if they are familiar with cases similar to your child's, and what exactly their fees will be. While many advocates have been through this process with their own children, be sure that your advocate has received the proper training from an organization such as Council of Parent Attorney and Advocates or Wrightslaw. According to SpEducational executive director and founder Lisa Mosko Barros, an advocate "can set you for success now and in the future" by "empowering families to understand the process and protocols so that over time they need me less and less."

This whole process feels overwhelming. Even with this information right in front of me, my head is starting to spin.

Mine too. Even after more than a dozen IEP meetings. I asked Lisa Mosko Barros of SpEducational what the heck we can do about that, and she had this to say: "There is so much onus on the parent to do the work. Even if you don't know the law, you know your child. You know if your child isn't being supported. I always tell people to create their community. Surround yourself with people who know more than you do. Be part of a support group or a resource group. Your child is entitled to a Free and Appropriate Education under federal law (IDEA). Your child has a legal right to FAPE. Trust your gut. Keep pushing until your child gets what they need."

Finally! We've settled the IEP! Now what?

Congratulations! Now, sign the IEP and return it. Be sure you keep a copy that's signed by you and all appropriate district personnel. Remember that if you want to call an IEP meeting at any point, for any reason (for example, amending goals, services, or placement), you absolutely have the right to do so.

What Worked for Me

- Talk to other parents or professionals who have been through this process.
- Make a list of questions and concerns—about my child, the school system, the IEP process. Ask school staff for answers in advance of the IEP meeting.
- Brainstorm and **write down** what I believe my child needs in order to receive a Free and Appropriate Public Education (FAPE).
- Identify and meet with a local lawyer and/or advocate. Be sure to get full information on their fees and process. Bring questions, concerns, and my view of what constitutes FAPE for my child. And always put all of this in **writing** and bring it to every meeting.

- **Schedule** the IEP meeting. For the annual IEP meeting, be proactive and schedule it months in advance to get a day and time that works best for me. Remember that parents can schedule an IEP meeting at any time, for any reason.
- If a school that I am not familiar with is offered in the IEP, visit the school before accepting or refusing the offer, and write down observations (see the template that follows). If I (or my lawyer) need to make a case for a different school, this documentation will be hugely helpful.

Expert Insight: What Do I Need to Know About IEPs?

Check out the Appendix for full conversations with the experts featured here.

Valerie Vanaman

Valerie Vanaman is a special education attorney and managing partner of Vanaman German, LLP.

- The goal is to achieve an acceptable outcome that delivers FAPE for your child.
- If there are issues or if it is contentious, meet with a lawyer at the first signs of concern.
- You need to be willing to make it clear that you want the hard answers—you do yourself a disservice by not hearing both the best *and* the worst.

Markeisha Hall

Markeisha Hall is a special education advocate and IEP coach.

- Create a vision statement and build goals that will get your child there.

- Think about how your kids can access everything in the whole school day.
- Your voice and what you have to contribute has weight, just as much as everyone else's.

Letter to Myself: Erick Puell

Dear Erick,

Today, as you begin your journey as a special education teacher, I wanted to say: Relax, you got this! I know you're anxiously waiting to meet your students and hoping everything will run smoothly. Spoiler alert, it won't. But, that's okay.

Here's what I need you to do: Focus on the students. Many times, the students coming into your early childhood special education program are evaluated in unfamiliar environments, and the evaluations may not reflect what the student's needs or strengths will be in your classroom. Use the IEPs as a blueprint. But always listen to your students. They will teach you everything you need to know and in turn will make you a better teacher.

You will become amazing at interpreting your students' needs, sometimes immediately, others with time. You will create many support groups for families, and establish inclusion clubs at school sites to help create awareness of all students with disabilities on campus. In doing so, you will help establish a more accepting school community. School personnel and students will see how amazing your students are.

Shortly after starting your teaching career, you'll become a father of two fabulous boys. The youngest will be diagnosed with a genetic disorder called Noonan syndrome, a condition that prevents typical development in various parts of the body. This often causes short stature, café-au-lait spots throughout the body, heart defects, and physical and developmental delays. At first, you'll cry, blaming yourself for being the cause of his condition. You'll worry about his future, whether he will be accepted by others or bullied at school. You'll have a 504 plan to address his needs at school to prevent him from being "benched" during recess for asking to go to the bathroom so often. You'll need to have medication at school to address his headaches and frequent nose bleeds. All of which will work out just fine. But your biggest fear is whether he will be able to live a long and normal life. When you are faced with those emotions, know that you won't be alone and you will work your way through them. There are plenty of people in your life that will help get you through it. Embrace those difficult moments. You will learn from them. The experience will make you a more efficient and empathetic teacher for your students and their families. I do, however, recommend that you start putting aside some extra cash for the future. There will be plenty of medical procedures for your child, all successful, but expensive.

Now don't worry, both of your children are excelling in life. Your oldest will surprise you with his talents and intellect. Your youngest is funny, strong, charismatic, and is great at sports. Know that both will surpass your expectations, thanks to how you and your wife raised them. Believe and trust in what you're doing. It pays off.

In closing, I wanted to wish you a great first day. Your students are going to love you! Although many won't be able to tell you that, trust me, they'll show you.

YOU GOT THIS.

Me/You

Templates

Letter to the school district in advance of your IEP meeting (yes, send this before every single IEP meeting, in an email or as a hard copy)

TO: Assistant Principal (or Person Coordinating the IEP)
FROM: Daphne Smith, mother of Taylor Smith
RE: IEP meeting, dated 05/07/2024
Dear Assistant Principal,
I am writing in advance of Taylor's IEP meeting on May 7, 2024, in order to notify you of the following:
We will be audio recording the meeting. (Note: if that is allowed in your state.)
Attending from our side will be: Daphne Smith/parent, Norman Smith/parent, James Jimenez/behavior therapy supervisor, and Mila Miller/friend.
We would like to request all IEP-related documents and paperwork in advance of the meeting, including all evaluations/assessments, goals, and other relevant items to be discussed.
Thank you.

School Visit Worksheet

School/Teacher

School name, location

How long was my visit

Teacher name, how long teaching

How many classroom assistants?
How long have they been here?

What is the current student/teacher ratio? The maximum student/teacher ratio?

How many special education classes are there? Are they accessible for my child?

Did you meet the assistant principal? Thoughts?

What grade levels are served by the special education classes and/or program?

What would my child's day look like in a special education classroom? In a general education classroom? Split between special education and general education?

Notes about school/teacher

Students

How many students in the class?

How many boys/girls?

Ages of kids?

How many kids with 1:1 aides?

Are there kids similar to my kid?

Are there kids whom my kid would benefit from being around?

Notes about other students (you can't ask diagnoses or other personal information)	

Daily Routine

Hours	
Daily schedule	(write schedule on back or take photo)
How much morning time for meals and self-help vs. instruction	
Notes about routine	

Classroom

What is the curriculum? Name? Where do I get a copy? Is it specific to special ed? Who at the school adapts it for special ed?	
How often can I observe?	
How sterile/inviting? Choking hazards? Clean?	

Size of room? How steep are ramps to get into room? Are there ramps?

How's the lighting? Any windows?

Restrooms: How far? Shared with other classes? If so, what age? Is changing table inside of a closed-door private restroom? Are toilets private and have a closed door? Will my child be able to access them with or without adaptive equipment?

Notes about classroom

Related Services, aka Therapies

For pull-out therapies, where is the room? How far from class? Will that take away too much class/therapy time to get my kid there?

Can I meet the OT, PT, and SLP?

How often do the OT, PT, SLP come in and work with the entire class? What is the schedule and duration?

If my child needs AAC (Augmentative and Alternative Communication, aka a device for communication), who on your staff is trained in AAC?

Notes about therapies

Playground

Outdoor space: How far from classroom? Surface (Concrete? Uneven? Shade?)	
Can my child access/reach/use playground equipment?	
Size of outdoor space? Does it get crowded? Would it be unsafe?	
Notes about playground	

Parent Questions and Concerns

Teacher, classroom staff, administration	
Classroom space and accessibility	
Outdoor/playground space and accessibility	
Schedule	
Curriculum	

Safety	
Inclusion opportunities	
Other students, crowding, socialization	

Template: Vision Statement Example

Mary will graduate from high school ready for a self-determined life of choice, including meaningful participation in the community, with rich opportunities for socialization, meaningful relationships, contributing to the community, and pursuing her interests. This may include employment or further educational programs, with minimal support to succeed. Mary will be able to fully communicate with both familiar and unfamiliar people, will be literate, and will have fine motor and gross motor skills on par with nondisabled peers. Mary will be able to independently perform hygiene routines (including being fully continent), will be an oral eater, and will be a very stylish dresser. Mary's goals in school and across service delivery areas will work in conjunction with this vision statement to serve Mary in achieving her optimum future.

Ask Yourself

- Do I understand how to get my child evaluated for an IEP?
- Do I need to seek clarification on the IEP process from our school district in order to truly be an equal member of the IEP team?
- What parents do I know who have been through the IEP process? What questions do I have for them?
- Does my school district offer IEP education/information classes?
- How can I involve my child in their IEP process to the maximum extent possible?

Where Do I Start?

- Schedule the IEP meeting.
- Notify the school who will attend, that you'll record it, and that you are requesting all relevant documentation in advance.
- Schedule a lawyer and/or advocate meeting if you'd like.
- Bring to the IEP meeting:
  - Your questions in writing
  - Your copy of the IEP
  - A recording device (fully charged)
  - A notebook and pen
  - Snacks
- After the IEP meeting:
  - Take the **unsigned** document home, read it, get clarification as needed.
  - Meet with your lawyer/advocate if that's your thing.
  - **Sign** the document and **return** it—**only** after you are certain you fully understand it and that it gives your child FAPE (that is: you are satisfied with what the IEP provides and/or you have contested parts you disagree with and those issues are resolved).
  - Breathe. You did it!
  - Now, mark your calendar to schedule your next IEP meeting in a year.

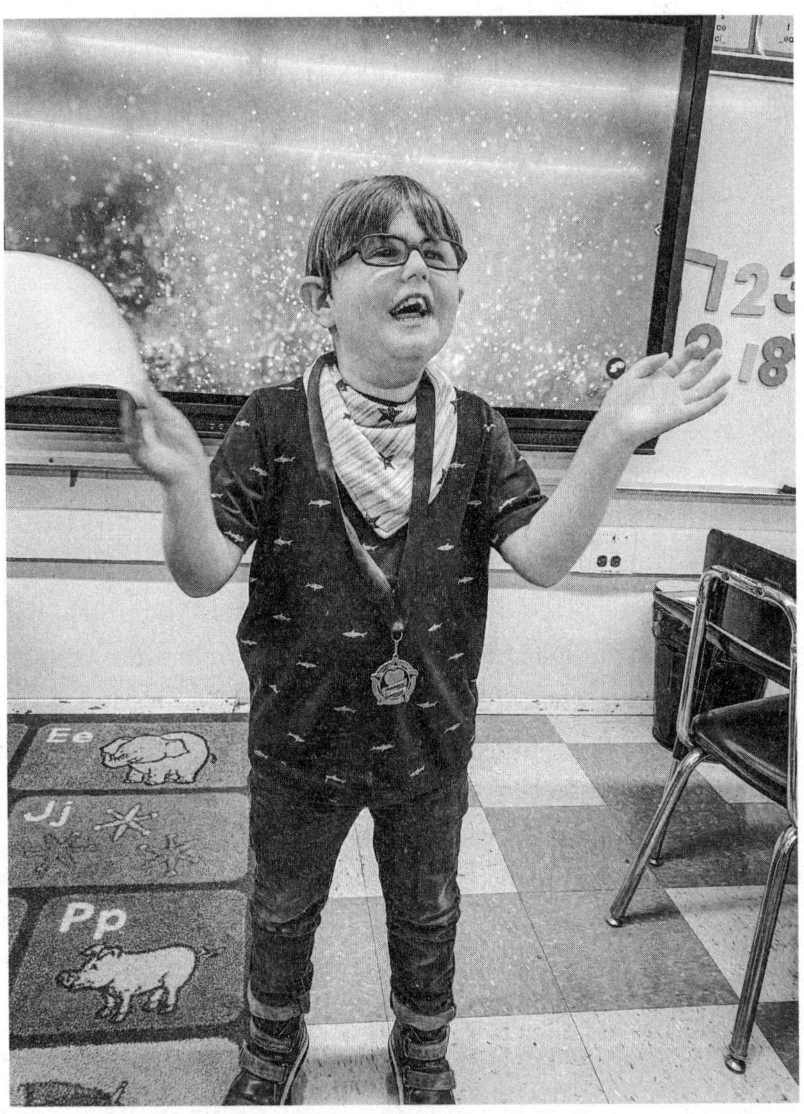

Image description: An excited boy stands in his classroom, wearing a gold medal around his neck, holding a certificate. Behind him, a screen with the image of gold confetti.

Photo credit: Andrea Casillas

CHAPTER SEVEN

Everything No One Tells You About School

The kid in that picture? Yeah, that's my kid. And I'm incredibly proud of him. He looks like he's delivering his acceptance speech at the Oscars or standing atop an Olympic medal podium. But what he is in fact doing is accepting an academic award in second grade. This was Aaron's first academic award. I totally cried when I saw that he had won an award for Digital Citizenship, even though I had no clue what that was.

When it came time to send Aaron to school, I was nervous. What if he doesn't like it? What if he's not learning? What if he doesn't make friends? But it turns out school is a place where he thrives. At school, he is respected and supported by his teachers, high-fived by his friends, and able to succeed as his unique self. His teachers have centered his days and his lessons on the things he *can* do rather than starting with the things he can't do yet.

As I mentioned in the previous chapter, it's not Unicorn School. But it is a public school that works for us. School looks different for each kid, regardless of their abilities. We explored our options, and while I had hoped to enroll Aaron at the public school in our neighborhood, that ultimately wasn't the right fit. I wanted him at a school that had both disabled and nondisabled peers, including peers with similar support needs to Aaron's. I wanted teachers used to teaching kids with needs like his, teachers who could genuinely educate, and not just manage, him. For us, inclusion looks like Aaron spending time with peers of all abilities, including kids who are also disabled. For Aaron, splitting his time between a general education class and his Special Day Class (SDC, aka special education class) has been a great fit. He transitions enthusiastically between classes, and he is welcomed by the other students. For other kids, spending their full days in a general education class or a special education class is a better fit. How did we know what to choose? We gathered our information. We took our cues from Aaron and adjusted accordingly. Even from a young age, we've made Aaron a part of the decision-making process. While there is much that he cannot communicate with words, because he is able to express his likes and dislikes, it was clear when he felt comfortable and happy about a school. With that in mind, we took a leap of faith. We do that a lot. We're good leapers.

As you prepare to send your child to school, trust yourself and your ability to do right by your child. We've had to switch schools in the past, and you might need to do that as well. Or maybe not. Work on what you can control, and learn from what you can't. It's not about everybody earning a Digital Citizenship Award. It's about empowering your child to succeed exactly as they are.

Speaking of that lofty award, I did figure out what it meant. Next to a grinning yellow star, it says: "Aaron loves technology! He is great at using it to participate in class and asking for what he wants. We love his big smile when he gets to use any kind of technology in class."

Guys, that's *everything*. My kid has figured out that he can communicate with his AAC (Augmentative and Alternative

Communication device, aka an iPad with a communication program). He can hold a stylus and trace letters. He can wait his turn to use it. All of this took years. And you know what? He *does* deserve an award for that. It's not just a pat on the back—it's an acknowledgment of who he is, what he can do, and that his teachers are seeing his personal progress as success. *That* is what I was looking for in a school for Aaron. Sure, a farm with goats and chickens would have been nice. But I'm thrilled with what we have found for him: a school where the teachers understand how to teach him, with students who are used to hanging out with disabled peers, and where Aaron can truly be himself.

The Basics

What will my child's school day look like?

This varies, depending on the school, the class, the curriculum, and the child. Ask your teacher for a copy of the school schedule. If your child is splitting their day between a general education class and a special education class, be sure to ask when the splits happen.

How can I be sure that my child will be appropriately supported at school?

Communicate with the school staff, especially your child's teacher. Be nice. Be helpful. Donate tissues and hand sanitizer and glue sticks to the classroom. And talk to your child, regardless of their level of communication. Communication will increase (and communication doesn't have to be speaking), and school is often the catalyst.

Full inclusion? Split? SDC? How do I know what's best?

This varies for each kid. When in doubt, err on the side of more inclusion and see how your child does. It is generally easier to scale back toward special education than to add more time in an inclusive setting. Consider if your child needs a one-on-one aide in order to access their education in a general education setting. The law is that your child should be placed in the least restrictive environment (LRE) for them to access their education. That means that all students have the right to be fully included, with appropriate supports, in a general education classroom.

How can I be sure that my child's IEP is being implemented?

Yet again: communication for the win! Your IEP will have goals that you can use as benchmarks for discussions with your child's teacher and service providers. Observe or volunteer in the classroom. Schedule time with your child's teacher, even for a brief check-in.

If I have concerns, do I have to wait until our next IEP meeting to make changes?

Parents can call IEP meetings at any time for any reason. You should let the staff know why you are calling the IEP meeting, and ideally have a sense of your goals for the meeting so that you can have a productive discussion of what's working for your child and what needs to be changed.

What if my child is outpacing their goals?

Congratulations! As an equal member of the IEP team, parents may suggest amendments or changes to the child's goals. Discuss with your child's team if an IEP meeting is necessary to reevaluate goals.

How do school therapies (aka related services) work during the school day?

Related services specified in your child's IEP will be scheduled into their school day. You should speak with your child's teacher about the schedule for these services, including how long the sessions will be and how many times a week your child will see the service providers.

Will my child be graded in the same way as their nondisabled peers?

The curriculum that has been agreed upon (in your child's IEP) will inform how your child will be graded. Children can be on a general education curriculum or on an alternate curriculum (intended only for those students for whom a general education curriculum is not appropriate). Your school can explain the grading system for your particular child.

If my child is in a general education class, how will they be taught and not just managed if they have significant support needs?

For many students, an IEP or a 504 plan will specify any accommodations that need to be made in order for your child to access their education. Some students require a one-on-one aide or other supports in order to access their education. Ideally, your child will be placed with a general education teacher who has the training and experience to best support your child. Be sure to ask your child's teacher: "What can I tell you about my child that will help you to best support them?"

What if my child is the only one in their class with their diagnosis?

This might happen. It always happens with us. We have found that it's less about a diagnosis and more about an IEP with the appropriate supports and ongoing communication with the teacher throughout the school year.

I'm still nervous. Should I just start my own school?
Probably not. But maybe. Parent Kristen Gray did just that. Kristen and her husband founded The Gray Academy in order to create the most appropriate learning environment where their disabled daughter could thrive. "We started The Gray Academy because there were no other choices. We're able to do what the children need at the school. Our teachers are all trained in working with kids with significant support needs. It feels like a community, and not an institution, for kids whose needs can't be met at a traditional school. Our school is able to integrate the kids' disabilities in a meaningful way. Is starting a school hard work? Yes. Is it impossible? No."

How can I prepare my child's teacher to best support my child?
Communicate your child's likes, dislikes, and motivations. I recommend that you create an introduction page that describes your child (check out the profile template in this chapter). You can give this page to your teacher and any classroom aides at the beginning of each school year. This is great shorthand for your child's teachers, as well as a way for you to document your child's progress from one year to the next.

What Worked for Me

- Listen to, appreciate, and support my child's teacher. Trust that the teacher can do this.
- Send my child's introduction page on the first day of school. Make copies for all of the classroom staff.
- Ask the teacher how I can support my child's learning outside of school.
- Schedule teacher conferences when needed. Listen. Ask questions. Ask how to best support the teacher in supporting my child.

- Connect with other classroom parents to share experiences and ideas.

Expert Insight: What Do I Need to Know About School?

Check out the Appendix for full conversations with the experts featured here.

Julissa Zamudio

Julissa Zamudio is an elementary school special education teacher.

- Every child is capable of learning. You just have to find their way.
- Teachers and parents need to take the time to find ways to communicate.
- You want what's best for your child, and so does your teacher. Become a team.

Dina Marie Swann

Dina Marie Swann is an elementary and middle school inclusion facilitator.

- Ask how you can ensure your child is getting everything they need to meet their physical and medical needs, as well as their academic and social needs.
- Be a partner in your child's education. The more involved you are, the more accountable people will be, the more collaboration you will have.
- Your vision for your child's future may be the thing that determines placement and goals. What is the future you are fighting for?

Letter to Myself: Rachel Ulriksen

Dear Rachel,

By the middle of kindergarten, Kevin's aggressive behavior at home and school was completely out of control: hitting, kicking, punching, spitting, biting, screaming, sometimes for no discernable reason at all. He attacked our animals and broke our possessions. His aggression carried over at school. And every time I was called. Sometimes three times a day. Despite everyone's best efforts the situation got worse, and worse, and worse. Because his chromosomal disorder is so rare, there was no way to predict if the situation would improve.

Then came the day I really started this journey in earnest. I walked to school for pick up, and the moment I saw the school building, I knew something was wrong. Parents were congregated outside, concerned. "It's just a lockdown drill," they told me. But, when I saw the school psychologist peering out of her window right at me, I knew it wasn't just *a drill.*

The school psychologist gestured for me to come in through the side entrance. She led me to her office, offered me a chair and a box of tissues, then took my hands in hers. "It's bad," she said. "It's the worst we've seen." Kevin had demanded iPad time. When his teacher reminded him it was time for math, he kicked her, pulled her hair, then pulled down his pants and tried to urinate on her. He had headbutted the aide, and nearly knocked her out. Gripping my hands almost too tight, she said, "I'm sorry Rachel. I'm so, so sorry." I'm crying now, remembering her face at that moment, but I didn't cry then. I guess I was in shock. I said, "It's okay. I'm okay," even though it wasn't and I wasn't. I was ready to break. I remember saying to myself: "This is a nightmare. You'll live through this fear and shame and pain—you'll do it for your two girls who are counting on you. But you'll wish you didn't have to live anymore. Nothing is ever going to get better."

That *was my beginning. I want to walk backward in time, into that office, and hold Rachel in my arms the way I would my daughter. I want to say:* Cry, my love. Don't hold this in, it will poison you. Let your heart break. True courage isn't holding yourself together, it's allowing yourself to fall apart. If you allow yourself to fall apart, you can rebuild yourself starting from this moment.

I know you think this is forever, but you're wrong. Everything is going to get better starting now. The change will be painstakingly slow, but a year from now Kevin will be a completely different child. You're going to find the right therapist, who will collaborate with you and with the school to create a plan. A plan that works for Kevin. You will visit a developmental pediatrician who will prescribe medication for Kevin's aggression. I understand you have reservations about that, but you have larger reservations about him being sent away to a school for aggressive children, as some are suggesting.

The next year will be filled with seemingly endless therapy sessions, countless failures, and oceans of tears, but by September, instead of getting three calls a day from the school you'll be getting three calls a month. The boy who avoided his neurotypical peers will gradually start to show interest, and by December will be spending half his day in the general education classroom. By spring Kevin will be named Student of the Month. When you get to the library for the ceremony, his entire school team, including the school psychologist, will be there to surprise you with balloons, cupcakes, and a card that reads "You did it!" You did do it—along with your amazing son.

I can't tell you it won't be a long road with a lot of mud and nasty bumps, but I can assure you it leads somewhere beautiful.

And I hate to say it, but that road could have been a lot shorter and less muddy if you hadn't wasted so much time being ashamed. I know you are afraid to admit what's happening because people can be mean and judgmental, but the world is filled with kind, loving souls who would have helped you along that road if only you'd admitted you needed a ride.

You have **nothing** to be ashamed of. This is **not** your fault. You're doing the best you can with what you have. Let people in. You can't carry the weight of this by yourself. Tell the truth. Tell it to anyone who will listen. When you find the courage to open yourself up, so much goodness comes flooding in.

Yes, there will be regression. You'll go months with no negative behaviors at all and then, **pow!** he's kicking you in the shins or pulling the dog's tail because you said no to a third cookie. You'll be terrified every setback is a portal back to this horrible moment where you're sitting in the psychologist's office wishing you didn't have to live anymore. Have faith. You'll always find a way to get Kevin back on track. Kevin is the best he can be because you were never willing to settle for anything less. He will go to school dances and be a camp counselor and perform in plays. He will win six gold medals for swimming in the Special Olympics.

In about five minutes the psychologist is going to come in here and tell you that Kevin has calmed down. She's going to hug you tight and tell you they're going to find a way to help him. This will open the floodgates and you will sob into this woman's shoulder for a good ten minutes. After you've dried your tears, she's going to tell you not to give up because she's not giving up and neither are his teachers.

This is not your forever, it's day one.

That's what I want to say to Rachel.

And to all the parents out there like me, I want you to know that nowadays when Kevin has a bad day, I refer to it as a drill. Drills are frightening at first when that piercing alarm sounds out of nowhere and you're not prepared. Then, when you realize what's happening, you just go through the motions. It's annoying, inconvenient, and unpleasant waiting for it to end, but it's not frightening because you know it's not real. Everything is fine and everyone is safe. It's just a drill, and any moment now the light is going to come back on, the sound will stop, and over the loudspeaker someone will say, "Good job everybody. You did it."

Love, Rachel

What to have at school for your child (bring everything that applies)

- Diapers
- Wipes
- Hand sanitizer
- Extra clothes: shirt, pants, underpants, socks
- Sensory supports: chewing toys, fidget toys, etc.
- Emergency contacts (yes, the office will have this, but best to have these in the classroom for immediate access, especially for children with medical concerns)
- Emergency information, including diagnosis, medical history, allergies, etc.
- Specialized supplies (for example, extra feeding tube supplies)
- Medications: to be kept in the office/with the school nurse, as per school policies. Be sure that school staff is versed on medication administration (including emergency medication administration) for your child. **Request and fill out the appropriate school paperwork before sending medications to school with your child.**

Templates

Parent Tiffany Stafford created the profile template on the opposite page for her daughter. Check out her blog for details on how to create your own free profile: our3lilbirds.blogspot.com/2017/05/how-to-make-one-page-profile-ellie-style.html.

Ask Yourself

- What does my child's teacher need from me in order to best support my child?
- Do I need to schedule regular conferences with my child's teacher?
- How can I foster meaningful connections between my child and the other children?
- How does my child feel about going to school? What cues can I take from my child in order to improve their school experience?

Where Do I Start?

- Create a profile for your child. Give copies to the teacher and classroom staff.
- Talk to your child about what their school day will look like.
- Connect with the parents of other children in the classroom.
- Enjoy a few hours of quiet. You've earned it.

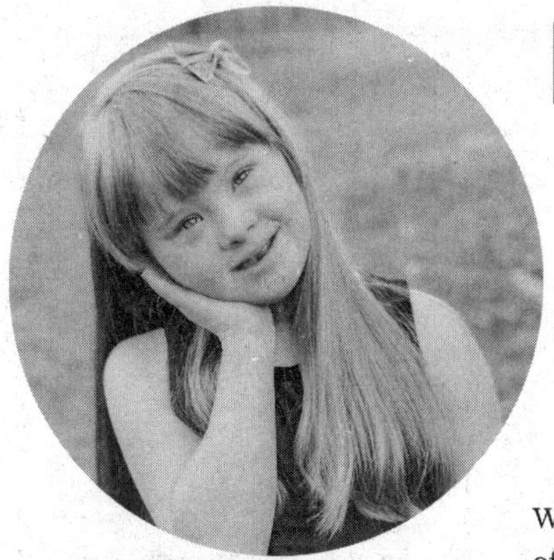

ELLIE STAFFORD
AGE 8
3RD GRADE

You can do it put your back into it.
-Ice Cube

VISION STATEMENT

We envision our daughter living a life of choice. We envision her being included in every aspect of life, including at school. In the future we envision her living a happy life surrounded by love and support.

STRENGTHS

- Visual Learner
- Reading on Grade Level
- Loves Spelling
- Social and Kind
- Funny
- Smart
- Fast Learner
- Excellent Memory
- Great Friend

WHAT WORKS FOR ME

- Peer Modeling
- Schedule and Routines
- First/Then Visuals
- Knowing Expectations
- Believing in My Abilities
- Praise Me for My Achievements
- Warn Me About Transitions
- Incentives
- Respond but Don't React

WHAT DOESN'T WORK

- Being Rushed
- Hovering, Let Me Try First!
- Reacting to Negative Behaviors
- Sudden Change in Activity
- Negative Talk
- Yelling
- Assuming I Don't Understand

WHAT I'M WORKING ON
(These are my main IEP Goals!)

- Successful Transitions
- Reading Comprehension
- Conversational Speech
- Writing Sentences - I Need Help Structuring Them

I LOVE: My Parents, My Brothers Will & Luke, Taco Bell, Dancing and Rap Music

Image description: A black and white one-page profile of a girl with Down syndrome named Ellie. Ellie has long blonde hair and smiles while resting her head in her hand. The profile heading is: Ellie Stafford, Age 8, 3rd Grade. Beneath the photo and heading, there are bullet point lists with the following headings: Strengths, What Works For Me, What Doesn't Work, What I'm Working On, and I Love.

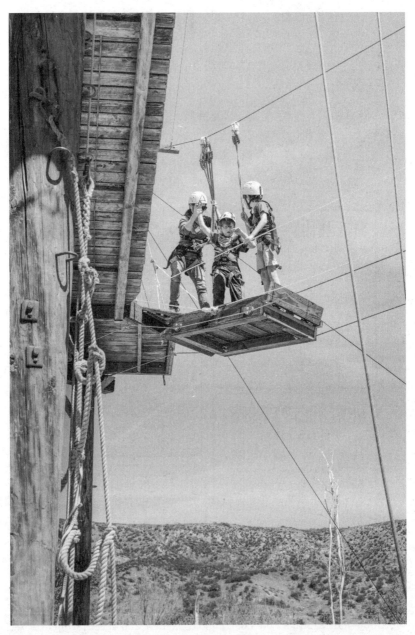

Image description: A mom and two children on an elevated, outdoor ropes course, stepping from one wooden platform to another, wearing helmets, in front of a blue sky.

CHAPTER EIGHT

Everything No One Tells You About Disability Rights and Advocacy

Is that Aaron on a ropes course? Yes, it is.

That looks really high up. Yes, also that.

It was as terrifying as you're imagining. Sean and I helped Aaron power through a fully accessible ropes course. Minutes before, we had watched kids in wheelchairs complete the entire course, zip line included, on their own. Before we found ourselves at The Painted Turtle camp, I hadn't even known that accessible ropes courses were a thing. It was wobbly and challenging and ultimately exciting and rewarding. The scariest part? Stepping onto that platform. The wood creaked like the porch of a haunted house. There was an amount of assistance Aaron needed to meet the challenges. But there was also an amount of it that he needed to do on his own. All of this frightened me. The doing it for him—what if I messed up and he went plummeting down to... oh, to the end of the safety rope. Sure, but even that scared me. The letting him do it for himself—what if he panics or just gives up? The figuring out when he needed assistance and when he needed to make sense of it on his own. When your child doesn't (yet) have the communication to tell you what they need, there's a lot of guesswork. That can be the most frightening part of all.

The uncertainty and the learning as we go have been a big part of our journey from the start. I find that I'm doing a lot of learning as I go when it comes to disability rights and advocacy, especially as I work on teaching Aaron to be his own advocate. Most of us don't come from the world of rights and advocacy, and it feels overwhelming to learn and to put into action. But here's the thing: when you're on a ropes course, you're essentially doing it alone; When you're in the world of advocacy, it's quite the opposite. All the information you need is out there. You just have to learn it. Because it matters. A lot. The more you learn, the more you will see how essential it has been that disabled people have led the charge for disability rights. Because that is who *should* be leading the charge.

So, where does that put parents, caregivers, and nondisabled allies? All parents start out doing everything for their children. Because babies can't shop for groceries. As parents of disabled children, many of us find ourselves in the lifelong role of parent caregiver. How do we embrace that role and also encourage our child's autonomy and independence to the maximum extent possible? What does that look like if our child's level of communication, interest, or attention span makes things like self-advocacy low on the list of preferred activities? I'm still figuring it out. My great hope is that my son will be able to advocate for himself, and that I will follow his lead and find the best ways to support the journey that he chooses.

Right now, here's what I know for sure: Listen to disabled people, follow their lead, and learn from their lived experience. As parents, it's easy to just do it all. It's scary to realize that there are parts of my child's life experience that I, as a nondisabled person, won't ever fully understand. It can be hard *not* to do all the things, especially when we have years ahead of us of changing diapers, ordering feeding tubes, charging AAC (Augmentative and Alternative Communication) devices, and hoping that Ikea never stops making the colorful little cups that are the only ones our kid will drink out of. Parents *want* to move mountains for their children, to be useful allies, and to get it right. Our roles can get blurred with the caregiving experience, and it can get really messy.

So, how *do* we get it right? We listen. We educate ourselves. We support organizations run by and for disabled individuals. We step back when others need to be centered. We ask how we can be useful, and we do those things. We show up over and over when we are asked. And we sit down when we are asked—better yet, before we are asked. Sometimes we even show our child that they can power their way through a ropes course. Because showing our children their power has to start somewhere. For parents, finding our power often starts with everything no one tells you about disability rights and advocacy.

The Basics

Why do I need to know about disability rights?

Your child's rights are not "extra" or "privileges" they're getting that others aren't. They're rights that your child is entitled to under the law. Don't let others make you feel like they're doing you a favor by building a wheelchair ramp into a classroom or allowing your child to be accompanied by their service dog in public. Those who require accommodations aren't getting something extra. They're getting equitable access. Disability rights are civil rights. They are institutionalized in federal law.

And what law is that exactly?
The Americans with Disabilities Act (ADA).

That's been around forever, right?
Nope. It was passed in 1990. The same year the movie *Home Alone* came out. So not that long ago. Many of us were alive at a time when these civil rights protections did not exist. Knowing the history of the disability rights movement shows both how far we have come and how far we have to go. For a primer on disability rights history, there are many great resources including the book *Demystifying Disability* by Emily Ladau and the movie *Crip Camp*, featuring disability rights leader Judy Heumann (both Ladau and Heumann are interviewed in this book). It was a *fight* to get the ADA passed, and getting it enforced is a fight that continues today.

What exactly does the ADA do?
In gigantic letters, the website of the Americans with Disabilities Act (www.ada.gov) states on its homepage: "The Americans with Disabilities Act (ADA) protects people with disabilities from discrimination." Right below, it goes on to say "Disability rights are civil rights. From voting to parking, the ADA is a law that protects people with disabilities in many areas of public life."

How does the law define disability?
The ADA website provides an answer to that in its Guide to Disability Rights Laws: "To be protected by the ADA, one must have a disability or have a relationship or association with an individual with a disability. An individual with a disability is defined by the ADA as a person who has a physical or mental impairment that

substantially limits one or more major life activities, a person who has a history or record of such an impairment, or a person who is perceived by others as having such an impairment."

Why doesn't it list specific disabilities? Why is it so broad?
According to disability justice leader Rebecca Cokley, "The power of the definition in the ADA is the big tent that it creates." She points out that there have been attempts to limit this, including in cases where the Supreme Court "narrowly interpreted the Americans with Disabilities Act's definition of disability." In response, the ADA Amendments Act (ADAAA) was passed in 2008. A (now archived) questions and answers page on the ADA website explains that this amendment made "significant changes to the ADA definition of 'disability' to ensure that it would be easier for individuals seeking the protection of the ADA to establish that they have a disability that falls within the meaning of the statute."

But my child has "special needs"! They aren't "disabled"!
Here's one of many great opportunities to learn from disabled adults. Disability advocates and activists have been vocal about using the word "disabled" and eliminating the phrase "special needs" to describe disabled individuals. According to Cokley, "The reason I always use the world 'disability' is because it's a word in law. It's a word that we as a community chose. Getting comfortable with that word is part of the armor you need as a parent raising kids with a disability. You can be very clear about what the law does and does not say."

Oh, so now you're the language police?
Nope, just listening to disabled people and following their lead. I hope people will follow my child's lead one day too.

Speaking of my kids, what about the laws that apply to school? Check out Chapter 6 about IEPs and Chapter 7 about school for information on the Individuals with Disabilities Education Act (IDEA). IDEA is a law that entitles every child to a Free and Appropriate Public Education (FAPE).

I don't feel like I can make a difference. I'm just a mom in Ohio working on my pickleball game.
The more disabled leaders I've spoken with, the more I've come to realize just how much this is everyone's job. In Ki'tay Davidson's acceptance of the White House's Champions of Change honor, he said, "I challenge the extent to which we place the responsibility for advocacy on those designated as leaders or 'champions.' Advocacy is for all of us; advocacy is a way of life. It is a natural response to the injustices and inequality in the world." It's okay to start small, to start in your community, and to start with advocating for your child's needs.

I feel like I need to know more. Where should I go to keep learning?
The ADA's website has lots of great info, as does the ADA National Network (adata.org). In addition, following disability rights leaders and organizations on social media can also connect you to people, information, and resources. Start online because it's easy, and that will lead you to opportunities to engage in person. You'll find role models for yourself and your children. I know I have. Judy Mark of Disability Voices United had this to say about the learning process for parents of disabled children: "Everything I learned in the early days was from other parents. Everything I learn today I learn from adults with disabilities. I've changed as a more sophisticated person and advocate. I take my lead from self-advocates. There is a degree of

self-advocacy that my child can do, but he can't advocate for systems change. For those who are disabled and able to advocate for systems change, they should be doing the arguing and we should be backing them up. We need to lead with self-advocates, and secondarily lead with family members. This is a hard road, but you and your child are not helpless or powerless. We can work within these systems."

What Worked for Me

- Follow disability leaders on social media. Read books. Watch documentaries. Listen, learn, repeat.
- Connect with disability rights organizations that support people with my child's disability (for us: undiagnosed rare disease, as well as other diagnoses).
- Begin to involve my child in self-advocacy by having conversations with him, bringing him to meetings from a young age (with appropriate accommodations).

Expert Insight: What Do I Need to Know About Disability Rights and Advocacy?

Check out the Appendix for full conversations with the experts featured here.

Maria Town

Maria Town is the president and CEO of the American Association of People with Disabilities (AAPD) and is the former senior associate director of the White House Office of Public Engagement during the Obama administration.

- The ADA was designed to provide rights and protections for as many people as possible. There is no hierarchy of disability or judgment of who is "disabled enough."

- For way too long, people with disabilities have been denied opportunities to speak for ourselves.
- Parents need to say that disability is hard so that their children have the skills to realize that the problem is not *them*, but that the systems they are confronting make things hard.
- We need to ask ourselves "How do we create environments for our kids to thrive?" We need to create spaces where everyone belongs as they are.

Elena Hung

Elena Hung is the cofounder of the kid-centered disability advocacy group Little Lobbyists.

- This *is* about the kids, so of course they should be front and center.
- We are changing the narrative by telling our children's stories. This is not charity. This is community.
- Always tie a personal story to the advocacy.
- It's not our child's disability that is the problem, it's the lack of support, the lack of services, the constant fight—*that* is the trauma.

Letter to Myself: AnGèle Cade

Dear AnGèle,

As of today, life will never look the same. Your baby Aundon was born prematurely, and your and Brandon's hearts will be tested beyond anything you thought was possible to endure. You know this already because of what you have already been through, and as rocky and earth-shattering as this new experience will be for you, remember this: love always wins.

You and Brandon will become fierce advocates for Aundon to ensure he gets the care he needs. Along with his doctors and the support of your village, you will be able to get to the bottom of his dying spells, make it possible for him to get the life-changing aortopexy surgery he needed, and learn how to meet his unique needs as an autistic child with a visual impairment.

It may come as no surprise to you that in Dubai, people with disabilities are known as "people of determination." This completely describes Aundon who has been determined to live, love, and have a space in the world since the womb. Due to your love and efforts, Aundon is now a teenager and has a heart and love that is so special. He always asks for hugs and lights up with such joy. He loves *being around his family and other kids.*

Because of Aundon's unique circumstances, he won't hit his milestones at the same pace as "other" kids. That's why it is important to celebrate the wins with every chance you get.

When he takes his first step, celebrate the win.

When he speaks for the first time, celebrate the win.

When he goes to the potty, celebrate the win.

When he communicates his feelings, celebrate the win.

What matters most is the progress he makes every single day. That alone is reason to celebrate.

Know that you can't do everything alone. It won't be easy. You will face the unknown frequently when it comes to Aundon's care, which will require decisions you won't immediately have answers for. Then on top of that, there will be numerous appointments that will need to be scheduled and kept track of, including IEPs, seeing his doctors, navigating with paraprofessionals, and working with his therapists.

Even your self-care stands to fall by the wayside when it is not intentionally prioritized.

This is why leaning on your village is so important for you, Brandon, and Aundon.

Who is your village? A whole host of people who are ready to show up to give care and love to all of you at every opportunity! These are the people who will gather around for a family meeting to find solutions to complicated problems and will jump at any chance to take Aundon to his appointments. These are the people that will take Aundon on playdates and create experiences in the communities that will forever be the fun times in his memory. These are the people that bring their world and families to join with you.

In addition to seeking help from your village, here is one practical way to stay on top of everything: Use a centralized digital storage solution to keep all of your paperwork in one place. Make sure you have many terabytes available for pictures and videos! For any family members who want to help out by taking Aundon to his appointments, you can share your virtual calendar with them so everyone can be on the same page. This will make it easier to coordinate everyone!

Beyond what you will do for Aundon, you will teach adults and kids alike that children like Aundon have nothing to apologize for. Children like Aundon will eventually become adults, and have so much to contribute. You will show everyone, even strangers, to treat kids like Aundon with compassion and genuine respect. You will awaken, and you will become aware that so much needs to happen for true inclusion to occur.

This will be especially important for Aundon as he gets older. Statistically, the odds are stacked against him. He will one day grow up and be at risk of receiving unfair treatment because history has shown that many people are unkind. As a little Black boy, he will be cute but as he grows up with his disabilities less evident, his responses and processing time may not receive the grace needed by authorities or communities if he is ever profiled. I know this sounds frightening, but there are steps you can take to ensure Aundon's safety. One way is by using behavioral therapy so he will know what to do and how to speak up for himself if someone asks him to be compliant in an authoritative manner when you are not with him. Another way is doing what you have already been doing: being a public advocate. These methods will go far and long to make sure Aundon and other children like him have a space in today's world.

Above all, I want you to remember that you are doing the best you can with what you have. Aundon will receive prognoses that will make you worry and people will give you advice you may or may not agree with. Remember you have a voice and it matters. Someone else's limit is not the perimeter that Aundon is restricted to. Ask the questions that need to be asked and don't be afraid to have lengthy conversations to get to the bottom of things. It's all about working from win to win instead of worrying about what's next.

Aundon is your teacher. The lessons that you will glean from him will be invaluable, not just for you, but for the world. His road map of lessons and love is a gift, make sure that you keep opening it to find every treasure from it. If you follow his guidance and listen to your intuition, you will find your path through everything.

Love always,
Aundon's Mom in the Future

Templates

How to tell your child's story in your advocacy

1. Center on your child and their personality, not just the diagnosis.

2. First tell about your child, then explain how a policy will impact your child/family.
3. Adorable photo.

Here's an example:

Aaron loves airplanes. He loves playing catch with the frozen peas at the grocery store, flashlight tag with his brother, and when other kids ask about his service dog. The California law against the misrepresentation of service dogs makes a difference in our lives, because having fraudulent service dogs out in public makes it harder for Aaron's service dog, Heddie, to do her job, which makes it harder for Aaron to fully participate in community activities. Please continue to support laws protecting legitimately trained service dogs. If you're lucky, you'll get to see Heddie and Aaron playing catch with the frozen peas in the grocery store someday.

Writing letters to public officials

In emails or actual mail letters (yes, people still send those) to your elected officials:

1. Keep the letter short. No one wants to read pages and pages and pages.
2. Introduce yourself. Mention if you are in the area that that official represents, or any other connection you have to the official. Did you vote for them? Donate to their campaign? Are you from the same hometown?
3. Clearly state the policy or issue you are writing about and your position on the matter, or the position you are recommending that this official should support.
4. Share your personal story about how this issue impacts you, your child, your family, and/or your community.

Reaching out to your reps via social media

1. Follow the social media accounts of your elected officials.
2. Like and comment on their pages and posts when you agree.
3. Share the posts of your elected officials that you like.
4. If you disagree, be constructive. Don't just be a jerk.
5. Include your district hashtag on posts to identify yourself as a constituent.
6. Tag your elected officials in your related posts.

Ask Yourself

- Do I understand the accommodations and access my child is entitled to under the law?
- What role models and organizations am I following in the disability advocacy world?
- Am I teaching my child to self-advocate? How can I involve my child in their own advocacy from an early age?

Where Do I Start?

- Learn the basics of disability history and rights.
- Seek out real-life disabled role models and peers.
- Follow disabled leaders and disability advocacy organizations on social media.
- Include your child in conversations, meetings, and advocacy any time their rights, accommodations, and future are being discussed.

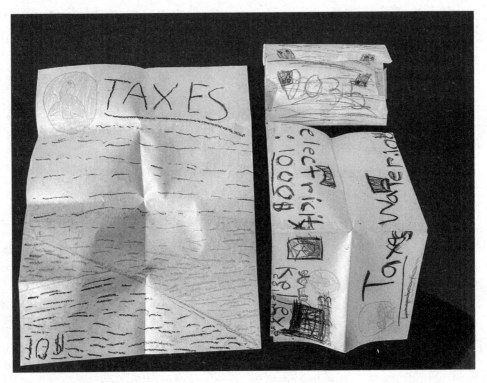

Image description: A child's hand-drawn crayon art of a tax bill and utility bills.

CHAPTER NINE

Everything No One Tells You About Financial Planning and Future Care Plans

Is that a tax bill and utility bills drawn by a seven-year-old?

Yes, it is.

???

Exactly. Welcome to my life.

When I picked Sean up from summer camp, he told me about art time that day. The kids had the opportunity to make something for their parents. I envisioned a macaroni necklace or a wood-burned plaque with my name on it, perhaps spelled incorrectly. Because I'm a mom and that's what we live for. When we got home, Sean could barely contain his exuberance. He'd made something for me! Something extra special! Something... uh, a tax bill? The look of confusion on your face right now is the exact look I had when I opened up the gift. Taxes? Sean couldn't stop laughing. Because taxes and utility bills are *hilarious*. Because, even as a seven-year-old at summer camp, you know that there's nothing worse than a stack of bills. So much for my macaroni necklace.

While the other kids were stringing beads and gluing feathers, my budding comedian made me this.

That was several years ago. I keep it in my To-Do folder to remind me that: 1) I need to teach my kids that paying bills and talking about money doesn't need to be scary, and 2) If my child drops out of school, he has a bright future as a third-rate comedian.

Why is it that so many of us find finances to be scary? Not just scary, but *scary*. First, there's the "women don't learn enough about finance" theory. We really need to do something about that. Then there's the "I'm afraid I don't have enough, so I'll just ignore it" theory. And the bonus theory for those of us with disabled children: "You mean I have to spend *how much* on that?" While most parents plan on their children growing up and supporting themselves, many parents of disabled children are faced with the reality that their children will need lifelong support—and that includes planning for their financial future and well-being even after we are gone. I've been quite seriously looking into becoming a vampire so I can live forever, but it turns out that comes with its own unique set of challenges, so I'm presently weighing my options.

That's why it's so scary. Because it kind of is. Don't freak out. Or do freak out. Freak out all you need to. Then read this chapter and make a plan. Every small step gets you closer to "Oh, that wasn't so bad," which is how we felt once we did our financial and future planning for our children. We sought out experts. There was no way I could have figured this out on my own. And the good news is that you don't have to either.

As with the "I'm neither a lawyer nor a doctor" disclaimers in other chapters, I'd like to remind you that I am not your financial advisor. I don't know how much money or debt you have, what your future goals look like, or if you're a fabulously wealthy vampire reading this chapter whilst mocking all us mortals. Only you know what is best for your family. Use this chapter to educate yourself so you can ask the questions to make the plans you need for your family to thrive. I promise it's less scary than a summer camp tax bill.

According to the National Disability Institute: "Researchers estimate that households containing an adult with a work-disability require, on average, 28 percent more income (or an additional $17,690 a year for a household at the median income level) to obtain the same standard of living as a comparable household without a member with a disability." There are the regular expenses, plus the future planning expenses, plus the things that pop up along the way. Our son wears through piles of rather expensive orthopedic shoes, and any equipment that includes the word "adaptive" suddenly includes some extra zeroes. And there's that wheelchair accessible van you've been eyeing…oh, and you left your job so you could be a full-time caregiver…yeah, it all adds up.…But, before you get overwhelmed by how you're going to pay for everything, first save yourself a boatload of stress and learn everything no one tells you about financial and future planning.

The Basics

Wow, Kelley, how do you know everything about this?

It's easy. I don't. I've sourced experts for our family's financial and future planning, as well as for this book. You don't have to do this alone. Educate yourself, and then seek out professionals who can walk you through the process and put everything in place for your family.

Do I really need a financial planner?

Probably. Do you know how to do this stuff? I sure don't. Remember that you'll need to have a plan that balances and works with government benefits, and that doing this wrong can result in a loss of government benefits for your kiddo. So, yeah, there's that.

Any financial planner will do, right? My neighbor Larry offered to do this for me for free.

That's very nice of Larry. You need someone who specifically works with disability planning. See that bit in the previous answer about losing government benefits. There's a ton to take into account. Most future care documents don't include information about caring for a service dog. Ours does. Yours will have loads of specifics that your child needs. You need a disability-specific planner, often known as a special needs planner, who knows how to plan for your unique situation.

I don't have the money to do this. And this stresses me out.

It *is* stressful. And everyone is coming at this from a different financial position. If your child has a social services coordinator, you can ask them to steer you toward resources in your state that work within your family's budget, even if you don't have any money to set aside for this part of the planning. Every state has a Council on Developmental Disabilities. The National Association of Councils on Developmental Disabilities can help you find yours. Or just google. I did. And I emailed a random person at our council to ask what people should do if they don't have any money for future planning. They emailed me back with resources and contact information in my local area. Hopefully your council will be as forthcoming.

How much is this going to cost me?

How much this costs will depend on what you're setting up and what your assets are. You can still make plans for your child's future, even if you do not have any assets. It's way less stressful to have this set up than not. Trust me. Start by having conversations with **disability-specific** financial planners so you can figure out exactly what your child's financial needs will be moving forward, how to utilize government benefits, and how to maximize your financial situation, both now and moving forward, including when you are no longer here.

I don't want to think about when I die. That's depressing.
Statistically speaking, you have a 100 percent chance of dying. Me too. Let's figure this out.

Okay, you have a point there. What is the bare minimum that I need in terms of planning?
My experts advised starting with an advance directive and a will. See the list of terms that follow to find out what exactly those are. I also recommend creating a person-centered plan (PCP). (Hey, look! There's a template for that in this chapter!). It's designed to guide your planning and keep it focused on the needs, goals, and vision of the disabled person. This will, of course, change over the years. Our son is ten now. When I was ten, my life's goal was to be the DJ at the local roller rink. I'm pretty sure his future vision will evolve, and I'm thankful that mine did as well.

What do parents forget to do?
Experts to the rescue on this one! Financial planner Shawn Francis said: "Parents or caregivers may be so busy with today that they fail to think of themselves, their own retirement, and/or life insurance." He provided a checklist for us parents that you'll find in this chapter's templates.

How much do I need to set aside for my child's future?

That depends on your family, your child, and your child's future needs. My crystal ball is in the shop, so I'll get back to you as soon as I'm able to see into the future again. You'll need to make a plan for finances into the future, as well as a care plan that details all necessary aspects of your child's care, especially those needs that they cannot communicate for themselves. It's a ton of work, but it gives you peace of mind to put it in place.

I don't understand any of this. I'm not a money person.

If you're an adult, you're a money person. Welcome. Many of us don't understand this, so let's start with some terms that you'll need to know:

ABLE (Achieving a Better Life Experience) account: A tax-advantaged savings account to which contributions can be made to meet the qualified disability expenses of the owner, or designated beneficiary.

Advance directive: A written statement of your wishes for medical treatment if you are unable to communicate them yourself. This often includes a living will.

Beneficiary: The person you name to receive your stuff, insurance money, etc. when you die.

Conservatorship/Guardianship: A judge appoints a guardian to manage the finances, affairs, decisions, and/or daily life of another person who is unable to do so for themselves. This can be the parent, or if the parent is not an option, another person may be assigned.

Estate planning attorney: An attorney who creates legal plans for what happens with your estate when you die.

Life insurance: Insurance that pays an amount to the beneficiary when you die. There are different types of life insurance, including term life insurance and whole life insurance. A disability-specific planner (often known as a special needs planner) can guide you to the right option for you.

Person-centered plan (PCP): A process for planning the services and supports that a person with a disability may need to live in the community, directed by the person receiving the supports.

Power of attorney: A legal document that gives another person the power to act on your behalf.

Social Security Administration: The government agency that provides monthly benefits (aka: money) for those who qualify. These benefits are known as Supplemental Security Income (SSI).

Special needs trust or supplemental needs trust: A trust that allows the trust money to be used for and by the disabled individual without this money affecting that person's eligibility for government benefits. Special needs trusts are intended to be used for expenses other than food and shelter, which should be covered by government benefits for individuals with disabilities.

Supplemental Security Income (SSI): A person's disability may qualify them to receive SSI benefits both as a child and as an adult. As of 2024, the maximum individual adult monthly SSI payment is $943. (I did the math and that's not much.)

Trust: A legal arrangement naming a person or a financial institution (that is: a bank) as a trustee, who holds and manages the assets (that is: money and all the other stuff) for the beneficiary (that is: the person getting the stuff).

Will: A legal document stating who will care for your children and how your assets (that is: money, house, car, pets, and all your stuff) will be distributed after you've died.

Okay, this is all starting to make sense.

Great. You've gotten your money's worth from buying this book. See, I told you you're a money person. Neighbor Larry will be proud.

What Worked for Me

- Just get started. Otherwise, it'll sit on a to-do list forever.
- Talk to my partner. Get clarity on our financial goals and future vision for our children. Involve our children to the fullest extent possible. Decide who gets custody of the children if we fall into a wood chipper.
- Talk to anyone named in our will and future care plan. Make sure they understand the responsibilities involved with being named as a caretaker of our children, especially disability-related responsibilities that they may not know.
- Create a future plan folder that contains all the information someone would need in order to support our children if we aren't around. It's not morbid, it's empowering. My kid likes to sing "Head, Shoulders, Knees, and Toes" before bed. If I don't write that down and he can't communicate that, how is anyone else going to know?

Expert Insight: What Do I Need to Know About Financial Planning and Future Care Plans?

Check out the Appendix for full conversations with the experts featured here.

Mark Solomon

Mark Solomon is a financial guidance specialist for families of disabled children, with a focus on helping families achieve financial security for both now and the future.

- You can't help anyone, and especially not your child, if you don't have a clear sense of your finances.
- Have a spot in your house with **all** of your paperwork.
- Start by knowing where you are financially. There is no shame in wherever you are right now.

Josh Fishkind

Josh Fishkind is the cofounder and Chief Operating Officer of Hope Trust, a technology-based trust company dedicated to servicing disabled individuals and their families with a full range of financial planning and future care planning services.

- It's nowhere near as bad to take care of this as people think it will be.
- Even families with really modest means need to consider how they're going to protect their loved ones.
- What does a future caregiver need to know that your child would not be able to communicate on their own?
- "Nothing about us without us" starts with empowering your child to be a part of creating their future plan.

Letter to Myself: Ellen Ladau

Dear Me,

Sonogram day! Daddy and I are so excited to see you, baby girl. I was hoping for a girl. Your name is Emily. "E" names just like me, your grandmas, and one grandpa. I have to pee so badly.

Looking at you on the screen is so amazing. Why is this taking so long? I really have to pee. Oh no!! Why is the technician going for the doctor? Is something wrong? Marc, I'm scared. It can't be Larsen syndrome; the geneticists said I could not, would not pass it on to my baby. What else is it? The doctor is taking so long. Then he said it: "Your baby does have Larsen syndrome." Shock, confusion, and sobbing. "The C-section will be more dangerous for your daughter," the doctor said. Call this doctor and go see this doctor. Daddy was strong for me. I went to the bathroom and then we went home.

My sweet daughter, this all happened this morning. I need to keep reminding myself that Uncle Jonathan and I have Larsen's and that you will be like us. I will know what to do. But will you hate me for giving you a disability, when deep down, despite the best genetic counseling, I feared there was a chance? Surgeries, braces, and social exclusion will be your future. I am crying as I write this letter to you. I really cried when I called Grandma Edie and Grandpa Harry. But you must know: I will love you with every fiber of my being and hope that you will return that love just as much. I will protect you fiercely and do everything I can to make your life even better than mine. Your entire family will love and support all of us as we start this journey. I really can't wait to meet you, Emily.

Love,
Mommy

Templates

Person-centered plan (PCP)

According to Tamra Pauly of Person Centered Projects, "Your goal is to get this read, usually in the room with your planners. Keep it simple and focused."

Your child's PCP should include:

- Name and birthdate.
- Date of PCP meeting.
- Changes in medical or disability status since the prior PCP.

- A future vision statement: Include both a short-term and long-term vision for your child, ideally crafted with as much of your child's input as possible.
- Your child's schedule: Include all school, therapies, and regular events.
- A section that addresses the following questions: How is your child currently being supported? What supports are they getting through school, insurance, etc.? Is this working? How could it be improved?
- A section that describes what supports your child needs to keep, or needs to have added, in order for them to achieve the goals and vision set forth in your future vision statement.

Goal sheet: finances

Thanks to special needs financial planner Mark Solomon for proving this template.

Short term (1–3 years)	**Midterm (3–10 years)**	**Long term (10 years +)**
Life insurance	House fund	Retirement savings
ABLE account	Car fund	College savings
Special needs trust (aka supplemental needs trust)	Vacation fund	Trust money
	Monthly total for goals: $XX	

Future care plan

What to include in your child's future care plan

- List of doctors and contact information and insurance

- Contact information for school services, social services, insurance, financial planner
- Where to access information on your child's finances and important documents
- Living situation
- Communication style
- Preferred people/relationships
- Preferred foods
- Preferred activities
- Aversive people/foods/activities/etc.
- Things other people wouldn't know unless you tell them

What goes into your box of important paperwork

- Future care plan (see earlier)
- Will
- Trust
- Insurance
- Power of attorney
- Birth certificate
- ABLE account or other accounts
- Government benefits documents and contacts

Organizing your finances 101

Thanks to financial planner Shawn Francis for providing this information.

Think of your household as a business. Any business has a balance sheet or profit and loss statement. What do you have coming in, what do you have going out, what is your profit? What do you do with that profit? That depends on your goals, income, risk tolerance, and other factors.

- Cash flow: How much is being brought in each month? Is there a need to earn additional income or cut expenses?
- Debt management and elimination: How much is going toward debt each month? What is the total debt? Is it manageable? What kind of debt (consumer or credit card debt, student loans, or tax debt)? What is the interest rate?
- Proper protection: What this means is having the right type and the right amount of life insurance so that your loved ones are protected when you pass. It is as misunderstood as it is vital. Ask yourself where you prefer to get your trusted information. Is it a professional, a company, or someone you have a relationship with? You can look into different types of life insurance, such as term, whole life, universal life, and indexed universal life. The best type of life insurance for anyone is the type that meets their objectives and fits their budget.
- Asset accumulation: Where are you growing your money? Is it someplace where the growth outpaces or remains competitive with inflation? Are you aware that there are financial products that can provide tax advantaged growth, such as life insurance? Aside from that, there are products or vehicles that can also protect your principal in a down market as well as give you income for life. Do you have 401(k) from a previous job that's at risk for loss? What's your risk tolerance? There are products that offer unlimited growth but carry a risk of loss, as well as those that offer principal protection. Does your disabled family member have benefits such as social security that may be impacted?
- Emergency fund: This is simply an account that consists of anywhere from three to six months or maybe even a year

of your expenses that's liquid (meaning that you can easily access the funds) **for emergencies only**. It's usually preferable that this account be protected against loss, such as in a savings account, but know that most banks offer rates of return that may not match the rate of inflation. Credit unions tend to be more competitive in that regard, but make sure to check with both to see what's available in your area.

- Estate preservation: This would include, but is not limited to, a will trust, a special needs trust, or the option that best suits your needs or the needs of your loved ones.

Ask Yourself

- If something happened to me today, are my child's finances and future plans in place?
- How much is my child able to be involved in these conversations and decisions?
- Has my child been able to participate in the decision-making process about their future care plans? If my child is not yet able to do so, how will I involve my child in this process in the future?
- Have future plans, wills, etc. been discussed with and understood by everyone named in our child's plans?
- Do I have short-term, medium-term, and long-term financial and care goals and plans that will secure my child's future?
- Have I taken into account all of the appropriate scenarios for the level of independence my child may have as an adult (if they will be able to support themselves, if they will attend college, if they will need residential care, etc.)?
- Do I have a binder of information that details my child's needs, specialists, routines, communication, etc.? Is this information with the person who will care for my child when I am no longer here?

Where Do I Start?

- Create a financial and legal plan: budget, will, trust, life insurance, power of attorney, and any other documentation you need to have memorialized.
- Create a future care plan notebook detailing necessary supports, contacts, doctors, preferences, etc. for your child.
- Create a person-centered plan with your child as involved as they are able to be in the creation of this plan.
- Assemble important paperwork together in a file: on your computer, a hard copy for yourself, and a hard copy for someone else to keep in case of emergency.
- Avoid wood chippers and/or research vampirism.

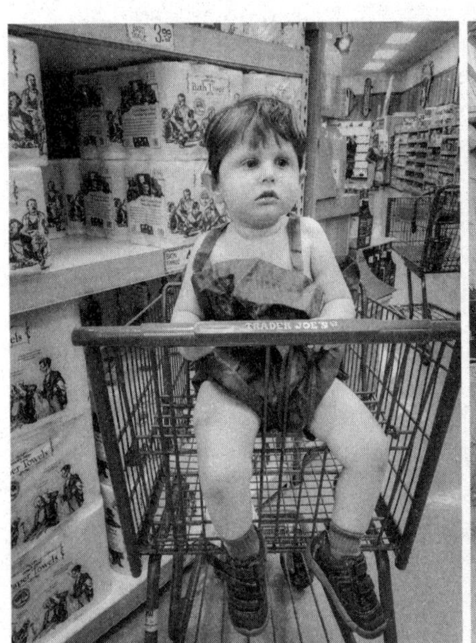

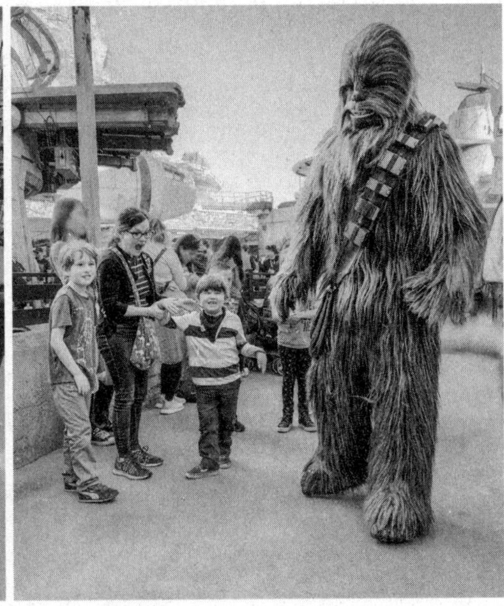

Image description: First photo: A male toddler with amazing brown hair sits in the front seat of a grocery cart, wearing shoes, socks, and a cloth grocery bag serving as overalls. Second photo: An excessively surprised mom wearing glasses and a striped shirt stands next to her two happy boys as Chewbacca casually approaches.

CHAPTER TEN

Everything No One Tells You About Inclusion in Your Community

Wait, this chapter gets two pictures?

Yep, sure does.

But won't the other chapters be jealous? Probably. We'll let them figure it out.

Community inclusion feels like something that warrants at least two photos. Because it's just that important. It's not always as easy as popping into the car and heading off to do a thing. When we do a thing, we also have to do a lot of things before, during, and after.

We recently took an overnight family road trip. Our packing list for Aaron included feeding tube equipment, feeding tube food, backup feeding tube food, meds, backup meds, supplements, diapers, overnight diapers, wipes, adaptive bed, adaptive stroller, loads of clothes and stylish bandanas, a stack of preferred books and toys and sensory supports, and all the supplies for Aaron's service dog, Heddie. Sean's packing list included an extra shirt and a toothbrush. I'm not sure if my husband and I packed anything for ourselves. It's a lot of planning, but we make it work. If we don't bring all of Aaron's food and feeding tube supplies, he literally can't eat. If we don't have his meds and backup meds, we could land in the hospital. If we don't have the book *The Snowy Day*, there's gonna be trouble.

And, speaking of trouble, that photo that looks like Aaron is wearing a grocery bag as overalls? Yeah, he's wearing a grocery bag as overalls. Desperate times, desperate measures. If you don't bring extra clothes everywhere you go, you too might find yourself getting creative and ripping leg holes into a stylish grocery bag. We spend a lot of time at the grocery store. Way more than you're imagining. Partly because, food. And partly because these routine trips have become a key part of Aaron's inclusion in the community. When he first started walking, he refused to walk anywhere else. So we'd show up before the magic doors opened (Magic doors! We love magic doors!), and the employees would say their good mornings as he walked laps around the produce. When he got older, we went there to practice safety and communication and service dog handling. One day when Aaron had an especially epic meltdown in the canned goods aisle, we laid down on the floor, and one employee walked up to us, said, "You and your kids are welcome here any time," and just kept going. *That* is how you let people know they are included. In recent months, Sean has taught Aaron to catch a bag of baby carrots, then take them back to our cart. We've also learned not to use a cucumber as a baseball bat for said bag of baby carrots.

Anytime we're out in the community, we can expect a range of reactions, from super awkward staring to "Could you please keep your child quiet during the movie?" to "You have a dog at the dentist!" Having a service dog has made people a lot nicer. Because dogs are awesome and we're the cool kids with a dog at the mall.

Way better than "Oh, you poor thing." We don't need your pity, thanks. But feel free to hold the door for us or toss us a bag of baby carrots.

Whenever our family leaves the house, we're on display. You can't not see us. One of us is probably squealing loudly and waving at every single stranger with one hand and holding his dog's leash with the other. Sometimes I do wish we could just blend in. But more often, I accept the challenge of teaching people about disability every time we leave the house. Most people don't have the opportunity to hang out with kids like Aaron. So when he's out, he's teaching them that disability isn't so scary after all. He's living his best life pretty much always. We're just along for the ride. And turns out it's a pretty great ride, whether it's standing on the sidewalk looking at airplanes or on a literal ride at a theme park.

We love ourselves a good theme park. Hence, Chewbacca. Chewbacca loves Aaron. Though I think Chewie is a little freaked out by Aaron's overly excited mom. Disneyland is where I first saw another kid out in public eating with a feeding tube. It's where we first saw a wheelchair user in a stage performance. It's a place where we just see other disabled people, like it's no big deal. Because it is no big deal. Because we're all just out and living life, regardless of what accommodations we may need. The accommodations aren't extra or some sneaky advantage. They're what my kiddo needs to access the world.

And that's what inclusion in the community is all about for us: access. Our son enjoys being a part of his community. So we give that to him. And we appreciate those who help to make it happen, whether it's the checker at Trader Joe's or a gigantic roving Wookiee. We've learned about inclusion by doing inclusion. And you will too. But, first let's talk about everything no one tells you about inclusion in your community.

The Basics

You leave the house with your kid???

Sure do. I've been surprised by how often people tell me that they never go anywhere with their child, that it's too much effort, that their child hates going out, or that they're exhausted by all the people out there who just don't get it. That's all a reality. Let's do what we can to make it easier on ourselves, to support what our children need, and to tell those people to buzz off.

Do you actually say "buzz off" to people?

And sometimes make an actual buzzing sound, yes.

Does it help?

It helps me. It frightens them. Everybody wins.

Do people really deserve that?

Sometimes they sure do. They stare. They lurk creepily as though I can't see them behind the toothpaste display. And the things they say…

They're just being nice. They want to say something helpful.

Let's be clear, it's not helpful to say "You know, my cousin's kid took this supplement and now he's cured!" while I'm in line at the zoo. Telling me, "Only special people get special children" kind of makes me want to barf. We're all "special people," no matter who our children are.

Do people get it right? At least sometimes?

More often than not, yes. I'm genuinely impressed by how often people *do* get it right. Kids are curious and ask questions. It's great when their parents encourage them to say hi rather than just telling them not to stare or to ignore us. I know you see us. It's cool. We find ourselves in many great and productive conversations with strangers, especially when we have our son's service dog with us. Everybody loves a dog.

Me too! I love dogs!

Exactly. Among the many benefits Heddie provides to Aaron, she changes his interactions with the world. When she's with us, people smile and start conversations. They talk to Aaron and ask him about his dog. Most people understand that service dogs are working, which means not to pet them. Please do be excited about service dogs, but also respectful that they're there to do a job, not to get belly rubs.

Does the service dog go with you everywhere?

Most public places, yes. She doesn't go to school with Aaron, much to the disappointment of his classmates and the PE teacher. She's come with us to theme parks, on airplanes, out to dinner, and is a regular at Aaron's inclusive soccer classes.

So, it's possible to go to a theme park with a disabled kiddo?

Absolutely. And most other places. Check out their website for disability access accommodations and plans. Call and ask if their websites don't answer your questions. Talk to other families who have been there. You may need to gather information, but once you do, please share your information with everyone you know.

How's parking?

Depends. And, if you need accessible parking, be sure you have your disabled parking placard.

How do I get a disabled parking placard anyway?

Google the keywords "accessible parking placard" (without the quote marks) plus your state name. For us, there was a form that our doctor had to fill out, which we sent in. Interestingly, this is the one place where I find the word "handicapped" used regularly. Let's make our parking "accessible." Oh, and our world please.

And airplanes—you do airplanes too?

Not often, but yes. Give yourself lots of time. The TSA Cares program can be helpful. Call the Transportation Security Administration (TSA) at least seventy-two hours before your flight: (855) 787-2227. They will assist you with making advance accommodations. For example, we travel with lots of liquids. It's helpful when TSA knows that in advance. Also, Aaron is a very enthusiastic traveler. That can look like lots of clapping and loud squealing. Cool. He's happy, we're happy. However, I get that strangers might freak out if they suddenly hear screaming mid-flight. See the templates section for the airplane blurb that we share with our flight attendants. We like to give them the language to be clear and supportive all at the same time. They don't need to apologize for our son's joy. They just need to let other people into our world. We often get extra cookies. Airplane cookies are a delight.

Wait, so you don't apologize if your kid is really loud on a plane?

We do a lot of *not apologizing.* If our kids are doing something wrong, absolutely. Ideally, they'll apologize for themselves. But so much of the way that Aaron moves through the world is just who he is. There's nothing wrong with it, it's just not how the average person does life. We made the decision that we don't want our kids to grow up hearing us apologizing for them when they're not doing anything wrong. It took some practice. But it feels really good. People react very differently when you cower and apologize versus when you say "Thank you for understanding." "Yes, that is my son blocking the whole aisle at Costco because he's dancing. Thank you for understanding. Want to dance?" And, quite often, people *do* want to dance.

My kid is unpredictable, aggressive, and might break things. Should I apologize for that?

This is a tough one. Your child may not be in full control of their body. Start with talking to other families in your situation. Many families face similar challenges and are afraid to talk about it. I've spoken with a number of friends who have said that for years they felt ashamed to talk about their child's aggression. Your child's challenges are very real and no doubt you're working hard to figure it out. Connect with other families, support groups, or therapists who have experience in this area. Safety is the most important thing, and there are people who can help you navigate it. The one thing I've heard over and over from families of aggressive children is this: Do not isolate yourself. There are people who will listen and people who are going through the same thing.

I'm nervous. Mostly about the staring, the comments, and just other people in general. It's a lot to feel like we're always on display.

It *is* a lot. For us, I've found it's helpful to remember that our interactions with the world have been overwhelmingly positive; however, there's always that one person...I find that it helps me to think through my reactions in advance so that I'm at the ready, don't get too defensive, and don't waste an opportunity to teach someone to do better next time. When people are staring at the feeding tube: "How cool is this—have you ever seen one of these before?" When people ask me to keep my kid quiet during a movie:

"This is quiet for him. Thanks for understanding." When kids are staring, I smile and say hi and invite them over. When adults are staring, I tend to creepily whisper "*I can see you*" and then they either say hi or scamper off in fear. Great.

When we go out, the world isn't necessarily accessible to my kid.
This can be a thing, especially for those with mobility devices and sensory support needs. Accessible playgrounds are increasingly common. And, if you poke around in your community, you'll likely find things like accessible/inclusive camps, activities, and even an Ultra-Accessible gem like theme park Morgan's Wonderland. More spaces are taking the concept of universal design into account—design that is accessible for everyone. Remember that whatever accommodations your child requires are not extra. Access is not an extra bonus. Access is equity.

But I can't find an inclusive activity program that works for my kiddo.
You might have to start your own. We did. As Aaron grew too big for the younger kids' soccer programs, we took a break. And he missed it. So we worked with the company that operated the soccer program to create an inclusive class geared toward kids of all needs, where siblings and the service dog joined, and families connected every week. It's effort, for sure. But for us it was well worth it.

Sometimes I just don't want to leave the house. I'm beat. I just want to sit at home and watch *DuckTales*.
Then, by all means, do exactly that. It's okay not to do all the things. Be honest about what you need—and sometimes that means you need to stay home all weekend. Sometimes that means you show up with the whole family plus a caregiver plus a service dog. Do you need to apologize for when you *just can't*? I'd say no. Rather than

apologizing, I find that a sincere: "I really appreciate you inviting us, but right now we need to lay low and watch *DuckTales*." If they respond with a "woo-oo," then you know they're your people.

What Worked for Me

- Follow my child's lead. He loves being out in the world. So we go out into the world.
- Know in advance how I will respond when people are not awesome or understanding. Know when I need to walk away, and when I need to correct the situation.
- Point out when people get it right. Send an email to Ikea about their helpful cashier or to the restaurant where the waiter escorted us to the accessible family bathroom.
- Seek out inclusive opportunities, such as camps and activities. Create inclusive activities if what my child needs doesn't yet exist.
- Bring the service dog everywhere.
- Have an actual packing list. Forgetting things can be a mess. Trust me.
- Research destinations in advance to learn about accommodations, safety, and nearby medical care.
- Call TSA Cares way in advance of flights to make a plan for accommodations in airports.
- Don't apologize for my child just being himself. Say thank you for being understanding or accommodating, and don't apologize for him doing things his way or for needing supports.

Expert Insight: What Do I Need to Know About Inclusion in My Community?

Check out the Appendix for full conversations with the experts featured here.

Christel Seeberger

Christel Seeberger is the founder and CEO of Sensory Friendly Solutions.

- Be as informed as possible about what the experience is going to be like.
- Ask your children throughout the day: How do you feel? What do you need?
- Set up yourself and your child for success with no apologies.

Paige Mazzoni

Paige Mazzoni is the CEO of Canine Companions.

- Service dogs are specifically trained to perform tasks for a disabled individual.
- The best thing you can do if you are considering a service dog for your child is to talk to service dog organizations to determine how your child could benefit.

Katie Griffith

Katie Griffith is the assistant camp director for The Painted Turtle.

- Look for family programming—it gives you the opportunity to see for yourself if your kids are ready.
- Many campers don't know someone back home who has their shared experience.
- Camp provides confidence, independence, and a sense of fun—every kid needs that.

Gordon Hartman

Gordon Hartman is the creator of Morgan's Inclusion Initiative, an organization focused on Ultra-Accessibility, which includes the world's first Ultra-Accessible theme park, Morgan's Wonderland, a sports complex, camp, Multi-Assistance Center, and more.

- It's about everyone coming together. It's not about "those people," it's about *everyone.*
- Inclusion can be a catalyst for changing culture.
- When you go somewhere, look around and ask: Is this Ultra-Accessible? Just think about it. Small things make a big difference.

Letter to Myself: Donna Lee

Dear Me,

My son has a disability... and so do I. Now what? That was my first reaction when, after several attempts to have him evaluated for behaviors that seemed different, he was diagnosed with ASD (autism spectrum disorder). Yet it didn't take me long to realize that I wasn't sad or scared or even disappointed. In fact, I was proud and happy... maybe even relieved that my son would have someone to relate to, having a disability.

Looking back, I probably assumed my lived experience as a disabled person automatically prepared me for parenting a disabled child. I got this, right? In some ways yes, and in other ways a definite no. There was a heavy pressure to serve as a role model, and at the same time, so excited that I could bond so deeply with my child. My experience was also layered with the fact that my disabled son has a nondisabled twin brother... and that I was taught, growing up, not to share or show my disability in public. Talk about inner conflict. Whether this was a cultural norm (coming from an Asian family) or an overprotective gesture, it clearly influenced my own unconscious bias when dealing with disclosure about my autistic son. Playdates, birthday parties, sports activities, family gatherings—every social setting gave me anxiety because I wanted my son to fit in with everyone else. I wanted to tell people that there was a reason he acted a certain way, but I also wanted kids to just be accepting of his unique personality. It wasn't easy seeing him get left out, but the negative scenarios I'd play out in my head were always associated with his disability. It took years before I would come to terms with my own internalized ableism and how I was applying this view to my son.

So I made a conscious choice to talk openly with my son, about his disability... about my disability... and how we could support each other. It was through these genuine, funny, insightful, and sometimes painful conversations that we encouraged one another. I can honestly say that no IEP (Individualized Education Program) could ever teach me as a parent how to create such a powerful bond with my child, understand his struggles, and come out on the other side with a way to navigate a world that is still not fully accepting of people with disabilities.

It was through our one-on-one sideline chats where my son became more self-aware as an autistic person. He's forged and strengthened friendships... and even figured out strategies on how to deal with conflicts.

One of the most important things I'd emphasize to my younger parenting self is not to become so overwhelmed by the barrage of evaluations, paperwork, terminology, goal achievement, etc. that you lose sight of, and connection with, your vibrant, loving, beautiful human being of a child. Find humor in the mishaps and truly appreciate the qualities that make your child so wonderfully lovable. Shift those ableist statements of "Don't do this or stop doing that!" to "How cool are you?" or "That's what I love so much about you!" That's the boost of confidence I wished I'd received throughout my childhood. It's the reason I hope and believe my son, now twelve years old, moves forward with independence, feeling empowered, and holding a perspective that being autistic is exactly what makes him fit in.

Love, Donna

Templates

Things people will say

Thanks to Effie Parks of *Once Upon a Gene* for sharing this handy-dandy bingo card to help you keep track of all the super unhelpful things people will say to you. I'd like to use my Free Space for things like "You're lucky to have such convenient parking!" and "My dog has seizures too!"

Things people say to rare disease parents

Bingo

Be glad they aren't talking, mine never shut up	They will grow out of it	Be glad they can't walk, mine get into everything	My kid wont eat either	God has a plan
Everything happens for a reason	Is your kid high functioning or low functioning	They always say Dad first	You aren't having any more kids, right	A feeding tube must be so much easier than trying to feed your kid
We don't allow any screen time	You child looks totally normal	FREE SPACE	I wish I could live day to day, I am too busy	Just you wait until...
Your child doesn't look that disabled	Isn't your child a little big for a stroller	You're such an inspiration	I could never do what you do	All kids do that
God only gives special kids to special parents	I don't know how you do it	Is your child retarded	What's wrong with your child	I'm sorry

@onceuponagene.podcast

Theme park checklist (that also works for zoos, museums, and loads of other places)

- Look online or call guest services to learn about their disability access accommodations.
- Download the park's app for maps, shows, access information.
- If your child needs an adult aide for support while in the park, will that aide receive free admission? If so, what do you need to do to make that happen?
- If you need to get a disability access pass in person, where will you need to go for that? Will there likely be a line or long wait there?
- Learn locations of accessible restrooms and service dog relief areas.
- Will your child need to transfer from their wheelchair in order to board rides?
- Will you need to use wheelchair accessible entrances to rides?
- Are there…
  - Quiet and sensory-friendly spaces
  - Assistive listening devices, captioning, sign interpretation for shows
  - Sudden, loud sounds
  - Flashing lights
  - Battery charging locations for assistive devices
  - Service dog relief stations
  - Wheelchairs available for rent, and can they be reserved in advance

Airplane blurb

When we fly, we hand a copy of this blurb to our flight attendants to read on the PA if they choose:

"We are excited to have a number of young guests with us today, one of whom may be expressing his enthusiasm for flying with loud or high-pitched squeals. We wanted to let you know that that's just his way of saying how happy he is to be here. Thank you for understanding, and may you have an equally joyful flight."

Ask Yourself

- What is my child's preferred level of participation in their community? What accommodations and supports do they need in order to be fully included? When do they prefer to be at home and/or in familiar environments?
- What is my child most interested in in terms of activities, events, places, people? Are these opportunities available in my community? Are they accessible? Do I need to create accessible opportunities?
- Is travel possible for our family right now? What would it take to travel for a day, a night, a week? What supports would we need to make that happen?
- What hesitations do I have about my child in the community? Are these legitimate concerns, especially for safety or health, or am I just getting myself worked up?

Where Do I Start?

- Learn what supports your child needs in order to have successful outings.
- Work with your child so they are fully included and participatory in everyday community locations, situations, and events.
- Plan outings in advance, including finding out accessibility information, accommodations, safety, and medical access. Think about what you would like to do in the next year, and make a plan for doing it that takes accommodations into account.
- Take your child everywhere they want to go.

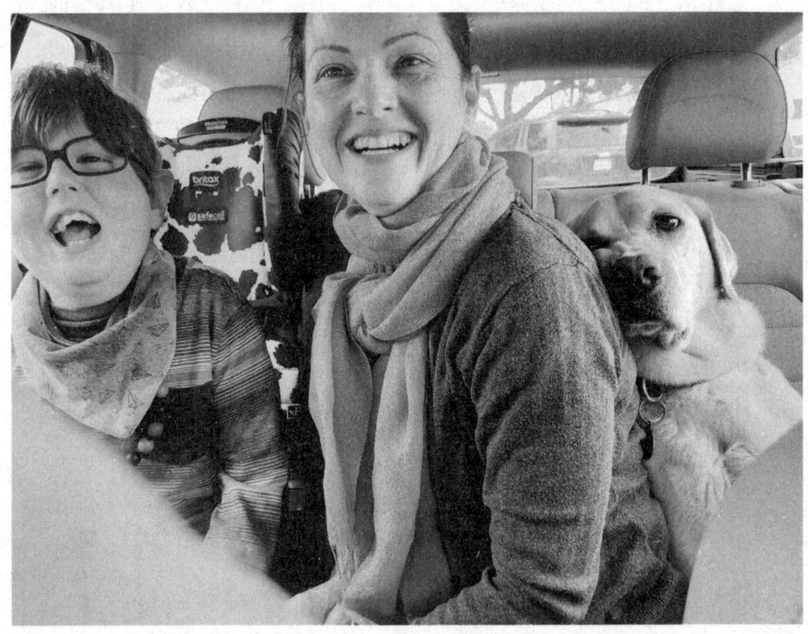

Image description: In the crowded backseat of a car, a smiling mom wearing a large scarf sits sandwiched between a laughing boy with glasses and a golden Labrador retriever lovingly smushing its face onto the mom's shoulder.

CHAPTER ELEVEN

Everything No One Tells You About What This Looks Like for You as a Parent Caregiver

Some days you're squished into the backseat of a car. Some days you're wondering why an emergency room visit takes ten hours. Some days you're in line for *The Price is Right* singing "Head, Shoulders, Knees, and Toes" with a group of total strangers. This life is never boring, that's for sure. There *is* a lot to love.

And, since I love a good metaphor, here goes: ocean kayaking.

I decided to try ocean kayaking in Channel Islands National Park. I had beautiful weather, a great guide, and unexpectedly strong wind, plus unusually large waves. Like *Moana*-inspired waves. At least that's what they felt like to me. I ended up way behind the rest of the group. No matter how hard I worked, I kept falling behind. Way behind. And I never got to take a break, even when I could see everyone ahead of me just sitting there and resting when they reached a calm spot in the sun. The more behind I got, the more the wind and waves picked up, and the harder it got. My goal went from "I'm going to catch up" to "I'm just not going to go backward." I literally sang the *Moana* theme several times. The guide came back to help me, and it just looked effortless for him, even as I was using every bit of my energy just to keep from going backward. It was 100 percent worth it. The views and the sea caves (sea caves!) and the wildlife (dolphins! sea lions! eagles! narwhals!) were amazing. I was proud of myself for making it through. But, at the end of the day, I was exhausted to my core, and on the ferry ride back, I fell asleep instantly while everyone else chatted and watched dolphins. And that is what it's like being a parent caregiver.

In my bright yellow kayak, I got everywhere I needed to go. I met supercool people. I was great at dodging rocks inside the sea caves. I saw the beautiful views. I probably appreciated them more than anyone else. But I had to work harder than anyone just not to drift backward. I had to get help that no one else needed. I knew that if I had stopped moving, I would have literally crashed into the rocks alongside a dead harbor seal. While everyone else was resting and having a snack, I never stopped moving. And, when I finally got to the ferry and *could* stop moving, I fell asleep instantly. I'm guessing I got more metaphors and thoughtful moments out of it than anyone there, but while I was working hard not to crash into rocks, I'll admit that I envied the rest of the group off in the distance enjoying their snacks. I would take the trip again in a second, even if I had known in advance how hard it would be. But, man, I would have loved to have had a few minutes when I could have just stopped moving. The view was dazzling at every point in the journey. I earned it. It was worth it. Just not relaxing.

Not relaxing, and also really hard. It's exhausting to constantly try to figure out how to do more and better and not to crash on the rocks or capsize into the very cold ocean. None of that takes anything away from the beauty of the day. I'd say it even amplifies it.

But, if someone wants to hear the story without hearing the hard parts (yes, there really was a floating seal corpse), then they're not hearing the full story.

And that's the thing with being a parent caregiver. It's *all the things*. It's the beauty and the triumphs and the surpassing expectations. It's the exhaustion and the being overwhelmed and the extra gray hairs. It's always wanting to do more and better while always wondering if you're doing enough. It's loving your child more than anything in the world, yet feeling totally inadequate and unprepared. Just like in the kayak, you figure it out. You sing the song from *Moana* a lot. You appreciate the views more. You go to bed way earlier. And you look for narwhals even if you know they're not there, because maybe today will be the day...

Parents too often feel ashamed or embarrassed to ask, "Where do I fit in?" when they've become a parent caregiver. We see stories online of other parents who take shiny photos where everyone is looking at the camera and appears to have recently bathed. We think about the path we thought we'd be on as we're changing our grown child's diapers. We wish we could have a conversation with our children because we want to know their favorite song or friend or flavor of ice cream. We wish they could tell us where it hurts. And none of this wishing takes anything away from how much we love our children. We need to be able to feel the feelings and to process them. We need to change the narrative from "I love you, but..." to "I love you, *and*..." I love you and this is hard. I love you and I feel alone. I love you and I want to figure this out for you and I don't know how. I love you and I love you and I love you. It's all part of the story. It's all part of everything no one tells you about what this looks like for you as a parent caregiver.

The Basics

Wait a second. You're saying it's okay for me to talk about all the things I'm feeling?

Not only is it okay, it's essential. Every person is going to feel differently about parenting, especially with children who have a range of support needs.

But I just feel crappy. And then I feel crappy about feeling crappy. I love my kid so much, but I'm seriously overwhelmed by all this extra stuff I have to learn.

That's a thing. It's a big thing, actually. This is something that I still feel and struggle with. I have two amazing kids. They're hilarious and joyful and fascinating humans. I've learned that I can still love and celebrate my kiddos exactly as they are while at the same time acknowledging that this is hard. We do ourselves a disservice if we pretend it's easy. Blending up food for a feeding tube is harder than grabbing a sandwich. Calling 911 on a Saturday night is harder than family movie night. Fighting the school district to get my child access to his education is harder than helping build dioramas of the Ice Age. The better we get about talking about the reality, the better we can get a handle on the reality. Hard isn't bad. It's just hard.

But you've got this totally under control, right?

Some days, yes. Other days, I feel like I'm falling apart and I can't find my glasses, which are probably on top of my head. Just when I think I've got it all figured out, along comes a curveball that knocks me out. I need to build in flexibility to all of my plans. I need backup plans for my backup plans. You'll probably need that too.

But these moms I follow on social media have it all figured out.
Do they? Stop believing what you see online. If it's making you feel bad to watch the Instagram version of someone else's life, maybe follow someone else or avoid social media entirely. I mostly follow people who build cool things out of Legos.

Good point. I think I'll start my own blog where I can be real about all the things.
Share your story! And remember that it's *your* story you're sharing—which means that, yes, your child may be a key part of that, but that they deserve dignity and privacy, so consider and reconsider posting their private life and information without their consent.

I'm on social media because I don't have anyone in real life who understands.
You might need to make some more friends. And that's weird, right? Yep, kinda weird. Until you do it, and it's a breath of fresh air to be around people who get it. I didn't realize just how much I needed to have friends who were also parent caregivers until they showed up in my life.

My partner gets it, so I'm good.
That's great. For real. Be sure you're talking with your partner about the caregiving experience; be sure you're honest about what's hard and what you need. Be sure you're communicating about everything, not just reading IEPs and medical forms together. When parents have different roles in the caregiving process, it's too easy to feel disconnected, especially if you're the parent who has given up a career or previous identity to be a full-time caregiver. It's a big shift.

Well, we talk, but not that much. That's a lot of communicating. Consider what conversations you're having in your head and what conversations you'd like to be having. Consider seeing a therapist, for yourself or as a couple. There's nothing wrong with working with a professional who knows how to handle *stuff.* Bonus points if it's a therapist with experience working with families of disabled children, or who identifies as disabled. Some even take insurance. You might need to try a few therapists before you find the right fit for you, and that's okay.

But I'm fine. I've got this. I can do this. Nothing is wrong here. I'm fiiiiiiiine.
Are you? There's this weird compulsion for us to say we're fine, even when we're totally not fine. Are you gritting your teeth as you're saying how fine you are? Are you feeling resentful that other moms are hanging out at the playground while you're looking for parking at the hospital? Are you interested in life and doing things for yourself?

Doing things for myself? You're kidding, right? I don't have time for that.
That's a tough one. You might not right now. But think about what you want to do, what is realistic, and what you want to work toward. When you're not working toward anything for yourself, even small stuff like showering on the regular, it's easy to lose yourself, and suddenly your life revolves around your child and their disability.

Don't all parents' lives revolve around their children?
It's different for each family, and it evolves as children grow. It can evolve very differently if your child has extensive support needs.

Will you be their caregiver for life? That's different than a typical parent-child relationship. If your entire identity is parent caregiver, is that the best thing for you, your child, your marriage, and your life? I talked to Lauren Clark, PhD, RN, FAAN, Professor and Shapiro Family Endowed Chair in Developmental Disability Studies at the UCLA School of Nursing, about this one, and she said: "The caregiver identity is a hard one. There's an expectation that parents will launch their children into an independent life. We are involved in webs of care for our entire life. Sometimes those webs are reciprocal, sometimes not. My job is to give as well as receive. We need to find ways for our children to be givers, not just recipients of care, and this changes how they participate in the web of support. You can find people of all abilities doing service, nurturing, finding ways to give. That's important to everyone's self-esteem."

Speaking of expectations, I'm from a culture with certain expectations and opinions of disabled kids. And some of those expectations and opinions are decidedly not awesome.

This can be a thing. Not with all people, and not with all cultures. But it's a thing. Maybe you're working on unlearning these ideas as well. Some cultures view disability as a punishment. Some families believe that disabled children should be kept hidden away. Cultural conditioning is real and it's messy and it's a lot to navigate. You or your family or your community may need to revamp long-held views in order to fully embrace your kid just as they are. Think about who you can trust in your community—and that can include your community leaders, fellow parents, and even your child's teachers. Speaking with a therapist experienced in navigating culture plus disability can be incredibly helpful to give you language and strategies to best honor both your culture and your child.

My friends keep telling me they're worried about me, and that I should take a yoga class. But I really don't want to take a yoga class.

I have those friends too. They mean well. But they're not you. You don't have to take a yoga class. Or go ahead and take twenty yoga classes. You get to choose. Early in my journey, I was getting unsolicited advice from everyone around me. I just wanted to scream, not to hang out in a quiet room with a bunch of bendy twentysomethings. I vented to my therapist, and she said something that really stuck with me: "Right now, your to-do list is your yoga." She was absolutely right. I needed to take care of business. I needed to get a handle on all the things. I needed this book, but it didn't exist yet. Eventually, I got around to yoga... and to writing this book...

Your to-do list? Seriously? But, that's not self-care!

Oh, the myth of self-care. I have opinions on this one. Why does self-care have to be an indulgent spa day or a wellness retreat? That might not be your thing. And that's okay. For me, self-care is waking up early and organizing my day. It's scheduling things that I look forward to doing. It's reading *A Series of Unfortunate Events* for the fifth time or wandering aimlessly through Target. Self-care is whatever brings me joy. Same goes for you.

Seriously? Your mental health sounds rather, um... off...

Yeah, I've been told that before. Nothing to be ashamed of. Mental health is real. There is absolutely no shame in wherever you are, in however you're feeling. I have friends who have been suicidal because they felt like they couldn't help themselves or their children (and I'm happy to report that they've found their way through). Mental healthcare isn't for broken people. It's for *people.* And you fall into that category, whether you just need someone to help you organize your thoughts, or whether you don't know how you're going to make it through today. Be proud of yourself for seeking help. You don't have to figure this out on your own. Call 988 to access free, 24-hour, confidential support (in English and Spanish) if you are feeling suicidal or are in immediate crisis. For those without insurance coverage for mental health, the National Institute of Mental Health can connect you with low-cost or no-cost resources in your area (see Appendix for further information). If you or someone you know is in immediate danger, call 911.

I'm also worried about my nondisabled kids. How is this going to impact them?
That's its own book. The impact varies with each family and each kid. Yes, this will have an impact on their lives. When I was interviewing Josh Fishkind of Hope Trust for the chapter on financial planning and future care plans, he spoke about his experience as a sibling: "This does impact siblings. It is a big factor in their upbringing and how they approach the world. Be aware that they will be impacted. How will they be impacted in the right way? Are they getting the right lessons, or just the stress? Moms especially are so focused on the needs of one child that it's easy for the needs of other children to get overlooked. It's a constant conversation and a tricky balance, but parents can work to focus on siblings so that the lessons learned will positively impact their lives."

Okay, so maybe I do need therapy after all.
Welcome to the club. High fives all around.

What Worked for Me

- Feel however I honestly feel. Don't tell myself I shouldn't feel a certain way.

- Seek out community.
- Ask myself honestly how ableism shows up for me, and what I can do to be anti-ableist in my own life.
- Schedule things that make me happy. Tiny things count (showering! Wordle! matching socks!). So do big things (overnight getaway!). Always have something on my schedule to look forward to.
- Be fully present in whatever I'm doing. If I'm with my children, don't worry that I'm not working. When I'm working, don't worry that I'm not with my children. Be where I am. Put down my phone.
- Communicate with my partner, let him know when I'm having a crap day/week/month, and be specific in letting him know what I need, even if that's just space.
- Figure out what it looks like to give both of my kids the support they need, schedule time with each one individually, and create meaningful activities together as a family.
- Figure out how much sleep I need (a lot). Do whatever I can to get that much sleep every single night.

Expert Insight: What Do I Need to Know About What This Looks Like for Me as a Parent Caregiver?

Check out the Appendix for full conversations with the experts featured here.

Amanda Griffith-Atkins

Amanda Griffith-Atkins is a marriage and family therapist, whose neurodivergent-affirming practice focuses on parent caregivers of disabled children.

- Parenting a disabled child often pigeonholes us into "that's my identity." So many parents, especially moms, start to lose themselves.
- Eliminate the expectation that we will reach mastery. This isn't something we reach the end of, and then we start the next thing. Mastery is not a destination to reach.
- Think about where you feel good, where you feel alive.
- The more we are honest, the more it blows the myth out of the water that we aren't allowed to have feelings.

Jessica Patay

Jessica Patay is the host of the Brave Together podcast, and founder of We Are Brave Together, an organization supporting mothers in the parent caregiving role through support groups, retreats, and resources.

- Caregiving moms often experience isolation and compassion fatigue.
- You don't need to be a martyr mom, with no self-care and no breaks.
- Mom guilt is real. And there's no need for it. Moms need to get logical about the guilt piece. When you have a child with a disability, the guilt can be exponential because the needs are exponential.

Don Meyer

Don Meyer is the founder of the Sibling Support Project and the creator of Sibshops (workshops and peer support for young siblings of disabled children).

- We need to honor the full range of experience. We need to validate siblings.

- The single strongest factor impacting a sibling's interpretation of their brother or sister's disability will be the parents' interpretation of the disability.
- The best thing families can do is to normalize the disability within the home.

Letter to Myself: Sarah Washington

Dear Sarah,

Everything will be okay.

You will grow. You will seek. You will learn. You, my beautiful, strong, capable mama, you will change. *You will be okay again.*

I am writing you twelve years from today to give you the wisdom I have earned and learned being Mary Elizabeth's mom. Your certainty, complacency, and "peace" about the world and its rhythms have disappeared. The world is now a cold, hectic, and sometimes cruel place that seems not to have noticed that your baby girl is hurt, that we *are hurting.*

I know that you are drowning in a sea of emotions right now. Those emotions will be there for years. You will become very good at recognizing and claiming these emotions. You are full of anger right now. It will turn into a hard burning RAGE—at God, at the world, at the evil systems left unchecked, at the fact that your precious baby girl has no control over her body, her brain, her life. You will be even angrier when you realize you have no control either. It was all an illusion. You will pray fervently for a miracle. You will even believe with everything in you that your daughter will be healed. And you will go to "healer" after "healer," hoping with each one that this *will be when she is made whole again. And then after all that work and hope, when she still has brain damage, the rage will come back... along with new feelings of betrayal, abandonment, disbelief, aloneness, helplessness, and absolute anguish that the God you have loved and worshipped and adored your whole life has not come in your time(s) of need.*

You will begin in the only way you know how right now: by DOING. Researching, searching, and finding anything and everything that may possibly help Mary Elizabeth. Your type A / Enneagram 8 personality (check it out!) will bulldoze forward for years, with urgency and energy that is ultimately not sustainable. You will become an expert in brain injuries, EEGs, epilepsy, stem cells, supplements, health and nutrition, G-tubes, suction machines, Russian goo, button covers, and so much more. What will make this life sustainable will be the beautiful people you meet who are on this journey with you. You will find common ground with people who your previous self would not have allowed in. They will share your pain: seeing our children suffering in pain, seeing the world reject our children, seeing how the world treats disability. And, eventually (it will take the better part of a decade), you will understand that the pain, anguish, and hopelessness is actually a place where we all become one. These are the places where we connect with humanity. These feelings are an inevitable part of the human experience. We lessen our suffering and others' by doing it **together**, *collectively, as* **one** *(mama) for all the kiddos (and* **their** *mamas) out there suffering. It is a way of staying connected even when you are so very clearly isolated.*

Your doing phase will shift after a very powerful experience with the **divine**. *I know you feel your experiences with faith and religion and God are mostly solid and good and full of hope. You are, to use your words, "on fire" for God. All this will change too. Being Mary Elizabeth's mom will humble you, literally bring you to your knees—sometimes daily for years. And in that one moment, in the spring of your daughter's second year of life, you will become forever transformed.*

You won't know what it means exactly or even how it happened or why, but you will feel the warmth and glow and beautiful fuzzy softness of the Holy Spirit, the Divine, the Ultimate Physician whispering sweetly in your ear, using the voice of a world-famous healer: "Everything will be okay."

Starting with that voice, the healing, and your own transformation, will start to grow. That delicious warmth will stay with you for months after, reminding you that God is with you—and you will learn to call upon IT when you are in the lowest of lows. IT will be there to breathe on you and in you, to envelop you, to hold you, and to pull you back up into the Land of the Living. And, years later, you will be able to recognize that God did *perform a healing that day: He showed up, planted the seed, and set in motion the healing of your mama heart. And, twelve years later, you will only sometimes wish He would've just healed Mary Elizabeth so life would be easier, more manageable, less painful, and more inclusive. Your old view of God, Christ, Jesus, the collective Church will be opened and widened to allow so much more light and love and true communion with others. Today, you are exploring the idea that maybe "this life" isn't a curse or even a mistake... maybe it* is *here to teach us how to communicate and connect and love in a different way. Mary Elizabeth is the teacher. She conveys joy, love, acceptance in a way that everyone is included.*

You will accept this journey, this life, yourself, your baby, and even your baby's cerebral palsy. She is whole and you are whole. For both of you, your value is simply because you are.

There is nothing to fix. There is only love. Your parenting experience will bring you to the realization that your capacity to love is unlimited.

Everything will be okay. Now go kiss that beautiful baby.

—Future Sarah

Templates

Thanks to Briana Mills, a licensed marriage and family therapist (LMFT), for the following lists.

Mental health checklist

- Am I feeling difficult emotions like grief, anxiety, depression, sadness, anger? Am I rarely feeling these, or am I feeling them often or throughout the day? Am I allowing myself to feel and express my emotions fully?
- Are my emotions interfering with my daily life?
- Am I finding joy and satisfaction in parenting, work, my relationship, my life?
- Am I relying on food, alcohol, or other coping mechanisms to make myself feel better?
- Am I eating, sleeping, and moving my body in healthy ways?
- Do I feel connected to others?
- Do I have things in my days and/or weeks that I look forward to?
- Do I have people I trust to talk to or help me with my feelings?
- Do I feel any resentment toward the tasks expected of me as a caregiver?
- Am I afraid to ask for help when it's needed?
- Do I feel like I deserve help if it's given?
- Do I feel like my role as a parent conflicts with my role as a caregiver?
- Am I setting boundaries when necessary to give time to my other roles such as spouse, parent, or self?
- Do I feel like my needs are often unimportant?

Remember that there is no shame however you are feeling, or in seeking help. If you feel that your mental health is compromised, seek the guidance of a therapist, talk to your doctor, and connect with those you trust.

Questions to ask a potential therapist

- Do you take my insurance? If not, what are your fees and how will I be billed? Do you have a sliding scale if I will be paying without insurance?
- What are your scheduling options? Are they weekly, biweekly, multiple times a week?
- Do you do telehealth sessions? Can these sessions be billed to insurance?
- What's the parking situation at your office?
- What is your cancellation policy?
- How long does each session last?
- Are you familiar with disability issues and/or ableism?
- I am a parent of a disabled child. Do you have experience working with my population?
- Tell me about how you work with your clients. Do you usually work broadly with clients over long periods of time, or do you set goals to be achieved over a shorter amount of time?
- Do you give your clients homework?
- What are your boundaries around contacting you outside of sessions?
- What is your approach to having conflict with a client in session?
- How do you view the therapeutic relationship?

Ask Yourself

- Do I have people in my life who understand what life looks like as a parent caregiver?
- Do I need to find a community of parents like me?

- Whose opinions and advice do I value and trust? Whose do I really need to ignore?
- What does self-care look like to me?
- Am I resorting to negative coping mechanisms? If I don't recognize these in myself, is there someone close to me who can be on the lookout for negative behaviors?
- Do I feel overwhelmed, anxious, depressed, or otherwise off balance? Would it benefit me to seek professional help?
- Do I know how to find the right therapist for me?
- How do I envision my life this week? This year? This decade? What are things I can plan for myself, outside of parenting?
- What brings me joy? How do I get more of that in my life?
- How am I working on the balance of caring for and supporting all of my children?
- What support do I need in order to best support all of my children?

Where Do I Start?

- Connect with organizations that support disabled individuals and their families.
- Join a parent group (online and/or in person).
- Make a list of things you enjoy doing. Schedule something to look forward to.
- Find a therapist for yourself. You'll be glad you did.

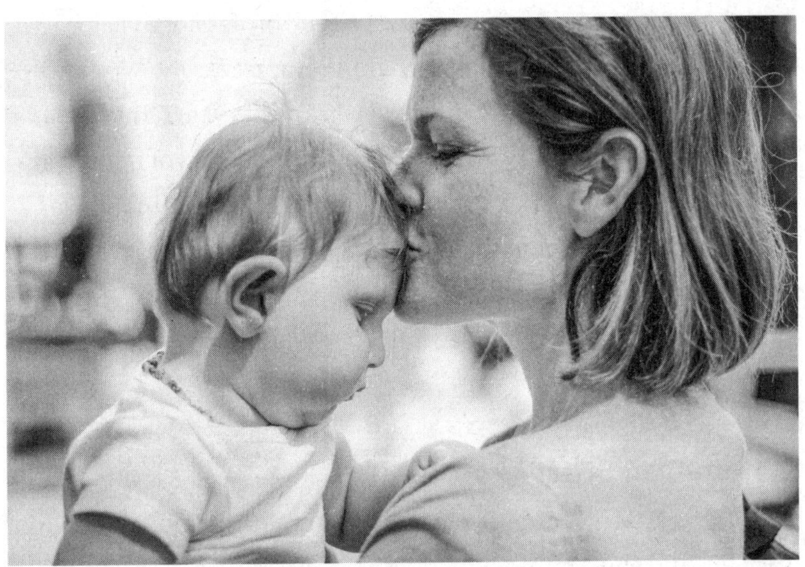

Image description: A side profile view of a woman with medium-length, straight hair kissing her baby, who leans toward her with his wonderfully chubby cheeks.

Photo credit: Eric Coleman

Conclusion

Well, that was a lot. I've realized that I use that phrase often when describing my experience parenting a disabled child, *a lot.* There are hard times and easy times, and amazingly magical times. There are ambulance rides to the ER, fights with medical supply companies, and watching our child spell his name on his communication device for the first time. My experience is exactly that: *my* experience. No doubt yours will follow a different path. Our kids are different, we are different, and all disabilities are different. But the things we most certainly have in common? The need for information. The need to not reinvent any more wheels. The need to spend less time doing the stuff, and more time loving our kiddos exactly as they are.

In the month leading up to turning in this book to my editor, I hit a wall. Aaron had a hard fall that resulted in a concussion and a badly broken foot, and I found myself sleeping in his bed for weeks to try to help him rest. Sean applied to middle schools, was assigned a giant book report, and built an elaborate leprechaun trap that took over most of our living room. Eric returned to working at the office (as opposed to a tiny room in our house) for the first time since before COVID-19. I found myself wildly underslept, finding and hiring a new caregiver, learning a new insurance policy, revamping most of Aaron's therapy plan, and moving mountains to prepare for both our annual IEP meeting and our annual Regional Center meeting (which landed days apart)—all with a book deadline looming. Severe weather alerts kept dinging on my phone, including flood warnings and evacuation alerts due to record rainstorms. Heddie the dog remained enviably calm and relaxed, and I probably asked her to fold our laundry at some point. This is what I mean when I say *a lot*. Because everyone's life goes through seasons where that's the case. The tricky thing I've found is that I'm in a season that just keeps going. I'll be a parent caregiver my entire life. There are things that will change and evolve; however, this role that I've found myself in is a role for life. I say that not as a good thing or a bad thing—it just *is*. And sometimes that role is hard. In writing this book and speaking with many disabled individuals, I heard over and over that, *yes*, being disabled is harder than not. Saying that isn't a complaint or a wish for something else. It's just a fact. There are just so many barriers, from the people who don't get it to the ramps that never get installed. And, as parent caregivers, we can acknowledge challenges without taking anything away from our love of our kids. Hard things aren't *bad*. They're just hard. Your hard is different from my hard. Because that's how life works.

What's universally hard for parent caregivers? All of the *stuff*. The systems, services, and supports that we all have to learn from the ground up, have to reapply for every year, and have to fight at every turn. It's hard for all of us. And there are so many factors that can compound to make the stuff even more overwhelming, challenging, and even impossible at times. Add bias into that and it gets even harder. Same ocean, different boats.

When I began writing this book, I had it in my head that I was writing it because I knew so much about the *stuff.* What I've realized is that I'm in fact writing this book because I will forever be learning the stuff. This book gives the most basic information so that you can ask better questions and make real plans for your child, your family, and yourself—real plans that involve your child in the decision-making for their own life as much as possible. I've literally been taking notes for myself as I've been writing. I even decoded our insurance benefits while writing the insurance chapter. Parenting a disabled child isn't a destination, or a game that you win if you just play your cards right. It's an evolving journey. It's educating yourself. It's celebrating every victory. It's laughing with your child while watching the dancing fountains—maybe for the rest of your life.

When I first brainstormed my list of experts to include in this book, legendary disability rights activist Judy Heumann topped my list. I had read her autobiography *Being Heumann.* I had seen the documentary *Crip Camp.* I laughed out loud watching her appearance on *The Daily Show.* I marveled over her decades of fighting systems and winning. It took me months to work up the courage to reach out to her. I did it after my submission to her podcast aired, alongside twenty-one other submissions, all answering the question "What does disability pride mean to you?" I emailed Judy. I heard back from her that day. She was enthusiastic about this book and emphatic about its necessity. She invited me to meet her in person at her home. We talked a lot about storytelling, about the story of the disability rights movement, and about her own story centering on empowerment, action, and lasting change. She ended our conversation by saying, "This is too important to stop now. When can you meet again?" We met again via Zoom, my kids made her Hanukkah presents, she sometimes called me at odd times with things she had forgotten to mention, and we had another date set to continue our conversations for the book. When I heard the news that Judy had passed away on March 4, 2023, I kept thinking about her vibrant smile. And about the tremendous impact her advocacy has had on the world, as well as on my family, and especially my son. Empowerment. Action. Lasting change. My phone dinged. It was a text from my friend Stephanie Bohn saying simply, "It's up to us to continue her work."

And it is. *All* of us. There is much that parents (both disabled and nondisabled) can do to support our children, to line up behind today's disability justice leaders, to ask what we can do, and to take action. My great hope is that this book gives you the headspace and the clarity to make the world a better place for your child, for your family, and, if you have the capacity, for the world. For me, this book always came back to one thing: *I'm not out to change my child, I'm out to change the world.* May you change the world as well. You might not have a choice. The world might not work for you or your child as it's built. So let's rebuild it. Challenge accepted.

Let's do this.

Ask Yourself

- What do I want to have in place for my child by this time next year?
- What big project can I take on first, and how do I break that into manageable steps?
- What is one thing I learned in this book that I can do *today*?
- Where can I go for further information that will benefit my child and our family?
- Who do I know who needs this information to best support their own child?

Conversations with Experts: Judy Heumann

Known as "the mother of the disability rights movement," Judy Heumann dedicated her life to being a civil rights leader and disability rights changemaker.

KC: What basics do parents need to know as they begin their journey parenting a disabled child?

JH: There's not one answer. It always depends on the individual child and the child's disability. It can even depend on when the onset of the disability occurs. There is just so much for parents to learn while they're also balancing life. What is important is for people to understand the disability, not just by a label, but with a deeper knowledge of disability, and the specifics of their child's disability and its manifestations. You need to go beyond labels. You need to dig deeper to find out what this actually means. You need to learn to set expectations for your children, and that might look different for each child. You need to find out what is there to help your child in their individual way.

KC: So many parents are shocked to learn their child is disabled. What can we do to take away some of that initial shock or fear or general mess of emotions?

JH: On some level, all families should be aware of disability and the resources that are out there. Even for those who are considering becoming parents, you need to realize that we don't know what's going to happen in any of our lives, in every area, including disability in children. There needs to be a basic acknowledgment that at any point during one's life, you could acquire a disability, have a disabled child, or your child could acquire a disability. Why does this matter? Because one of the most important issues is being able to **really think about what your views are**

of disabled people. In many ways, it's as important to have a mindset change as anything. We need to talk about how we take that journey, how we learn more, and how we grow.

KC: What would you say to parents who are struggling with their own internalized ableism?
JH: I'm a little cautious to jump to certain words, like ableism, when there is a bigger discussion to be had. That word can be appropriate, or it can be charged in a way that is not entirely helpful. In the case of a family member or close friend who truly loves this child, is it really ableism or is it limited exposure? It's complicated because *ableism is the reason* for such limited exposure to disabled people. If you are experiencing disability in yourself or in a family member, it's important to address the ableism, and also to know what your or their rights are. **The time when it's the most daunting is this period when you are figuring out what you need to do to start learning. It's about ableism, but it's also about a void of information. Why is there a void? Because of ableism.** It's all linked. The question is this: How do you begin to acquaint yourself with information that you need? You don't have to be a specialist in everything. You need to start with broad, accurate information, including how to connect with groups of disabled leaders and similar families. There are parent information centers in every state—and too many families have no idea. Organizations like Disability Rights and Education Fund (DREDF) and others have excellent parent programs. We just have to find the information that we need, and that can be a lot of work.

KC: How can families begin to access information that they can understand and use?
JH: Parents don't have time to do a lot of studying. Find what works best for you. There is material out there. It can be hard to

figure out. It shouldn't be, but it often is. In so many ways, systems are not set up to help you. So much can happen when you connect with groups. When I worked in Berkeley, we started a peer counseling group that paired parents with disabled adults. Think about how your child can meet others with similar disabilities. Peer support is very important for everyone. It's important to find other people you can learn from, even if they are not in identical situations.

KC: Too many parents don't know the basics of disability rights and protections. Where do we begin to educate ourselves?
JH: There's a need to have things reasonably and simply explained. When looking at the basic laws, look at why did these laws come about? IDEA and the ADA haven't been around for that long. There used to be nothing. IDEA and the ADA are in place to help remove barriers that have limited disabled people's ability to participate in society. They're about EQUITY. All of this presupposes that parents understand the concept of rights. But not all parents know that. How big is your book going to be? There's a lot to cover.

KC: How can parents begin to empower their children in their own advocacy?
JH: Think about assisting your child to move independently through life—with any child, disabled or not. From when your children are young, think about decision-making and expressing likes and dislikes. If your child is one year old, it will be very different now than when they are eight. If you haven't allowed your child to make decisions from an early age, everything will be different. Parents need to think of encouraging decision-making as part of supporting their child's development. **Don't discount your child's ability to speak up for themselves.**

KC: You've been advocating for disability rights for decades. Does it get easier?
JH: There are hard times all the time. You think you've got something good going, and then something changes and you're pulling your hair out. There will never be a time when all needs are going to be addressed by the system. You have to be an advocate for life.

KC: What's your secret? How do we raise our kids to be like you? I want my kids to be active, and empowered, and to love themselves exactly as they are.
JH: What I tell parents is this: Your children will look up to you as a role model. Teach them to question authority, to feel confident, to network. You need to teach them knowledge and expertise, but also not to be afraid to pick up the phone or to push when they need to. Prepare your kids to one day do this for themselves. There are hard times all the time. Don't just know the basic laws, get to the point of using your voice. We need to ask ourselves if we are looking at empowering our disabled children differently than we are empowering our nondisabled children, and if so, why? When I think about my parents, they didn't know anything about what was happening with me. They were immigrants. There were no laws. There wasn't anything. Period. We found our way. They taught me to be an advocate by using my voice. They taught me to find my voice. When we talk about my parents, what I think is unfortunate is that there are not enough parent stories. We need a breadth of parent stories so we can learn from one another. What you're doing with this book I very much believe in: allowing people to tell their stories. You may be in a family or community where they are accepting of a disabled child, they are going on the journey with you, they are helping you figure out what to do and how to do it. But in other cases, the journey is different, there may well

be biases against the child, or even a belief that the parents committed a sin that caused the disability. There are so many considerations, even within cultures and communities. All people have different personalities and different beliefs. **We need more people to tell their stories.**

Letter to Myself: Kelley Coleman

Dear Kelley,

You are right. Your baby was just born and you know that he is disabled. No one believes you. You'll shut down. You'll pretend you're not worried. You'll spend hours crying on the couch with your baby crying in your arms and your toddler crying in the kitchen, refusing to come to the couch because he knows he can't help. You fear that no one can help.

And that's where you're wrong.

It will take years before someone puts a name to how you're feeling right now. Inadequate. *Completely, totally, and in all ways inadequate. You feel like you have no control over your life, your future, and most importantly, your baby's health. Now,* that *you are totally right about. Right now, you can't control any of that. You'll do everything you need to do. Because you have no choice. Your husband will move every mountain he can. He will be amazing. But so much of this,* you *will have to do. It will be hard. You will become an expert in everything from neurology to complex laws to financial planning to the best industrial blenders. And even when you become an expert in all of this and more, you will still feel inadequate. You'll go to sleep every single night wondering if you could have done more.*

Could you have done more? I don't know.

But here's what I do know: This is so much bigger than you, this awful feeling that never quite goes away. You'll meet one person after another who is just like you, who is scared, who is overwhelmed, and who goes to bed every night wondering if they've done enough. You'll wish you could help their kids, just like you're helping yours. But you can't. *Instead, you'll do something even better. You'll teach others how they can do this for themselves. You can't change your child. You'll learn that you don't need to. What you will change is this awful feeling. You'll teach people where to start and how to do the things. You'll spend years swearing you'll never write this book. And then you'll write it.*

While you're writing, you'll realize that no matter where you have been in your journey, there is one thing that has been a constant that has gotten you through every single thing: You love this little boy. And he loves you. He loves his dad and his brother and waking up every single day. Even on the hardest days—and there are plenty of those ahead—everything takes a backseat to love.

There is always love.

Feel what you need to feel. Do what you need to do. And know that on the other side of everything, there is always love.

You've got this. I promise.

—Kelley

APPENDIX

Introduction

California Department of Developmental Services, Service Access and Equity

www.dds.ca.gov/rc/disparities/

U.S. Department of Education Office of Special Education and Rehabilitative Services

sites.ed.gov/osers/2021/08/osep-releases-fast-facts-on-the-race-and-ethnicity-of-children-with-disabilities-served-under-idea-part-b/

Chapter 1: Everything No One Tells You About Getting Comfortable with Disability

Experts

Rebecca Cokley

rebecca-cokley.medium.com

www.fordfoundation.org/about/people/rebecca-cokley

Oliver James

@oliverspeaks1 on Instagram, TikTok, YouTube, and X/Twitter

Emily Ladau
emilyladau.com
Podcast: www.theaccessiblestall.com

Parents

Christine "Chris" Tippett
raremomlife.com

Resources

Association of University Centers on Disabilities (AUCD)
www.aucd.org
Directory of state programs: www.aucd.org/directory/directory.cfm?program=UCEDD

Centers for Disease Control and Prevention (CDC)
www.cdc.gov
CDC disability statistics: www.cdc.gov/ncbddd/disabilityandhealth/infographic-disability-impacts-all.html
Increase in Developmental Disabilities Among Children in the United States: www.cdc.gov/ncbddd/developmentaldisabilities/features/increase-in-developmental-disabilities.html

Disability Visibility Project
www.disabilityvisibilityproject.com

Diversability
mydiversability.com

Ford Foundation
Disability rights: www.fordfoundation.org/work/challenging-inequality/disability-rights/

Helen: The Journal of Human Exceptionality
helenjournal.org

National Library of Medicine
www.ncbi.nlm.nih.gov/pmc/articles/PMC1449452/

Parenting Without Pity **podcast series**
rootedinrights.org/our-stories/parents/

United States Census Bureau
US Childhood Disability Rate up in 2019 from 2008: www.census.gov/library/stories/2021/03/united-states-childhood-disability-rate-up-in-2019-from-2008.html

Conversations with Experts: Rebecca Cokley

Rebecca Cokley is a disability justice activist, currently serving as the first US disability rights program officer for the Ford Foundation. She previously served as the founding director of the Disability Justice Initiative at the Center for American Progress.

KC: Disability is new to me. My child is disabled and I'm feeling alone in this.

RC: Just because disability is new to your family doesn't mean you're alone. Disability is in one-third of households. Eighty percent of kids with disabilities grow up in a household without anyone of the same diagnosis. You already know disabled people. They may not feel comfortable disclosing their disability to you, but I promise you they are there. Every state has a parent training and information center. There are tools and resources available in any language. Some days *will* be hard. It's okay to say that it's hard.

KC: My kid isn't that disabled. They're just "special."

RC: The word "special" needs to be banned. You won't find the word "special" in legislation. I always use the word "disability" because it's a word in law. It's a word that the community has chosen. You can discriminate against me because I'm "differently abled" or "special" or whatever the newest term is—but not because I'm disabled. Getting very comfortable with that word is part of the armor you need as a parent in raising kids with disabilities. For some parents, the internalized ableism is so strong that they won't tell their kid they're disabled. They'll go above and beyond to put the supports in place without ever telling their kids—and their kids end up feeling like they've been lied to for years. We need to use the word "disability."

KC: Big picture, I'm afraid of what disability will mean for my child. Does it automatically mean my child will be marginalized or discriminated against?
RC: Absolutely. No amount of education, no job, no country club membership, no anything will protect your child from ableism. It sucks. I was a presidential appointee and I still see it all the time. There is nowhere without ableism. Even within disabled spaces you'll deal with lateral ableism. It is the reality.

KC: That makes me angry. So much of this makes me angry.
RC: If you're not angry, there's something wrong with you. Be angry at the systems and the discrimination, not at your child's disability. Disability rights are civil rights. People have spent their lives fighting for the disability community, for your child's rights. There's a lot of work still to be done. It's okay to be angry.

KC: Some parents are hesitant to accept the expertise of disabled people in regard to their child. Why is that?
RC: Disability is so much more than a diagnosis. Often parents reduce disability to a diagnosis to feel safe. It scares parents that there are people who will understand their child, and that part of

their child, more than they ever will. That's not something all parents are comfortable with. Your child belongs to a different culture than you do. It's so important for you to have a community in real life of disabled people who your child can relate to. You want someone you trust who your child can go to. You don't want them going online and talking to strangers. You need role models for your children who can relate to their life experience. It doesn't take anything away from you as their parent. There will be conversations your child won't feel comfortable sharing with you. And that's okay. They need someone they can call. I'm not teaching my children to grow up to be me. I'm teaching my children to grow up to be themselves. That's not "parenting a disabled kid," that's just parenting.

KC: How do I teach my child to feel good about their disability?
RC: The most important thing you can do for your kids is to have real-life disabled friends who your child can relate to. I had adults in my life who reflected my experience. Teach your child that equal access is not extra, accommodations are not extra.

KC: So I should probably put up a social media page and talk all about my kid, right?
RC: Parents need to be careful about what they post online for any child. Do not post half-naked photos of your child online. Ever. Yes, there are predators, even in your parent groups. Conversations around boundaries and consent start at your child's earliest ages. Those conversations are even more important with disabled children. That doesn't go away if your child communicates with alternate means. Teach your kid about the rights of their body. As kids with disabilities, we are taught to let anyone touch our bodies. Teach them to say no. Teach them to push back. The right to own your body is a powerful thing. You learn that from your

parents. Remember that their disability is their experience, not yours. Think carefully about if you are putting your child out there in a way that they wouldn't want to be represented.

KC: When I grew up, I never saw disabled people in leadership roles—or anywhere really. Please tell me that's changing...?

RC: Historically, disabled people weren't listened to. They were put in institutions, locked up, sold to carnivals as entertainment acts. This is what we are working against—societal and legal attempts to keep us from having a voice in our own lives. We only recently have our first generation of elders in the disability justice community: Judy Heumann, John Lancaster, Justin Dart, Dr. Geraldine Hawkins, and others. These folks actually built the boat while sailing it. They spent their lives fighting to be deinstitutionalized, for their education, for jobs, for their rights. Because of them, our generation has been able to see disabled people as peers, as well as leaders. Our generation is broadening the definition of diversity. We grew up finally having disabilities represented in the media, starting with *Sesame Street* and *Mr. Rogers*. We watched Pedro Zamora on *The Real World* become a disability icon. With more disabled writers and creators, we are getting more and better disability representation in the media. We are seeing great examples of disabled characters, as well as real-life leaders like Tammy Duckworth and John Fetterman. Pop culture leads the awareness. Policy follows pop culture.

KC: I feel like I want to be a force for good. But this is a huge issue. Can one person actually make a difference?

RC: The disability rights movement needs everyone working together. Not just disabled people. Everyone. Greater awareness is growing. It takes people speaking out. It's not just about being included anymore. It's about thriving. Taking up space is radical.

It's power. Refuse to be quiet. Don't just try and conform. Spaces need to be inclusive. We need to reconfigure the world to work for everyone. Some families feel like they need to hide their disabled children. We can shift that by seeing disability normalized in society and in the media. Parents can start with including their child in everything in their community. They can teach their children to be unapologetic about who they are.

KC: What do you wish you could tell all parents—especially nondisabled parents—of disabled kids?

RC: Expect the unexpected. It's like parenting any kid. There are things that will happen in a typical course. There are things that won't. Allow your kid the flexibility to be human, and to make mistakes. Allow them to dream. Make sure they know there are options. Encourage them to pursue what they love. Have high expectations.

Conversations with Experts: Oliver James

Oliver James is a social media influencer and literacy advocate who rose to fame when he used his social media to chronicle his journey of becoming literate as an adult.

KC: How did growing up without an understanding of your disabilities impact you?

OJ: I heard "behavioral problems," or "dyslexic," or "learning disability," but the adults never really talked to me. They talked around me. You just sit in a room and they give you tests, and the next thing you know, you're put in a special class, and no one has explained to you what's happening. The biggest problem for kids is a lack of awareness. You need to know who you are.

KC: Statistically, Black boys are disproportionately labeled with behavioral issues. What would you say to Black boys who want to have a strong voice but are afraid to use it?
OJ: Find one person who believes you. Find one thing you love. Pursue that love with everything you've got. Other people do not have to like it. Find it. Hold on to it. That's the thing that will come back and save you. It can be sports; it can be deep sea diving. Put yourself in the space, even if there's no one in that space who looks like you. Create that space.

KC: You've spoken out about not feeling like you belonged in certain spaces as a child. How can we make sure that our children feel they belong in every single space?
OJ: Parents can give their children the gift of letting the world see who they really are. Your children belong everywhere. Be the role model for belonging, being in spaces, being yourself everywhere. If you show your child that they belong in the world, they will follow your lead.

KC: Do you feel there's a pressure for you to operate in the same way as everyone else who's not neurodivergent?
OJ: Yes. I'm not going to Yale. Yale doesn't have a place for people who don't read. My brain can't function that way. I have a different way. So I found social media. I can tell people the truth about me and I can win. I never thought I could be that. I thought I had to be somebody else. I'm not scared now. That changes the game for me. I always had the ability to do this—but now I'm not trying to do it like somebody else. Kids can watch my videos and say, "You're me."

KC: What would you say to parents who want to help their child succeed but don't know how?
OJ: Let your child lead. Don't just try to change them. Connect to your child by being part of *their* world. It may not feel right for you.

But you need to enter their world, to join them. Teach kids that they have a voice. My whole life, with my ADHD and learning disabilities, people were trying to stop me. I didn't know my genius as a kid. Let children learn about the things they love and they will show you their gifts. Put your own ego aside. Your kid needs you.

Conversations with Experts: Emily Ladau

Emily Ladau is a disability rights activist, writer, storyteller, digital communications consultant, and author of the book *Demystifying Disability*.

KC: Why should nondisabled people care about inclusion?
EL: If we believe in inclusion for everybody, that really does include everybody. It's about recognizing that an accessible and inclusive world is better for all of us. We should care about other human beings, not because we see them as charity cases or we're pitying them or see them as victims. Being inclusive creates access. For example, not everyone can get up and down a curb, but everyone can use a curb cut. Many parents don't have any experience with disability until they have a disabled child, but remember that you could become disabled at any time, so why wouldn't you want a world that is more welcoming to you if you are suddenly disabled? What if we all just accepted disability as part of the natural order of things?

KC: What does it mean to be an ally to the disability community?
EL: It's not a checklist you follow, and then you get a gold star. It's about **action**—the continued, meaningful action that you take. It's a journey, not a destination. There is no pinnacle of allyship. It's not a competitive sport. Allyship is something you do day in

and day out because you care about the humanity of people and you value their place in the world.

KC: "Nothing about us without us" is key to the disability community. What do parents need to know about this mantra, especially as it relates to being a nondisabled ally?
EL: Disabled people need to be leading the disability movement, activism, and conversation. That means that nondisabled people should not be speaking over disabled people or claiming that they know best for disabled people, and that can include you for your own child. Parents can sometimes view it as alienating when someone tells them that they don't know what's best for their own child. But it's important to center your child's preferences and life experience and to tap into your child's communication, even if they are nonspeaking. More broadly, a lot of parents take up the space where disabled people can take up space. You know what it's like to be the parent of *your* disabled child. Just like I only know what it's like to exist in my disabled body. The best thing to do is to advocate alongside us and with us rather than speaking for us or over us.

KC: How can parents build a community of disabled people to walk alongside?
EL: You can't start tokenizing. Don't expect any one person to be the expert on disability. We say there's a lack of disability representation—but there's also a lack of effort to find that representation. The reality is that it's actually out there, you just have to look for it. Take the time to seek it out. Engage on social media. Listen to podcasts. Read a book. Start somewhere.

KC: As a nondisabled parent, this feels messy. I don't want to claim disability as my own experience, but any parents' lives

are intertwined with their children's. How do I honor both my child's experience and my own?

EL: Live in the messiness. Things are going to be messy. Differentiate yourself from your child. You are not your child. Your child is not you. Yes, you as a parent are going to feel the pain of ableism, and you as a parent are going to feel distraught when you see your child suffering through a medical issue. That's real. Ableist attitudes can be directed toward parents. Here's an example: "How dare you bring this child to a play; they're making noises and they don't have a right to be here." Recognize that you are experiencing ableism through your lens as a parent, and your child is experiencing ableism directly as a disabled person.

KC: How can parents act in allyship without declaring themselves the Hero Parent who's here to be the savior of the disability community?

EL: There are people who take on the entire identity of Special Needs Super Mom! I think it comes from a place of love, but that it's also a coping mechanism. I wish that people would stop putting the entirety of their identity into their children in that way. Your child's disability isn't *your* life—but it gives a structure to your life. And it can change the entire structure of your life. You can find ways to separate your identity, even if the structure of your life is tied to your child's support needs. Who you are within the structure is still you. You were a person before you had a child. It's okay to take on a new identity, but it's a part of you without being all that you are.

KC: But this is my kid. I don't know how to do that.

EL: It's a challenging balance. A parent is coming from a place of being a parent. They're responsible for this individual. They love them. They want to see them succeed. Parents can feel discounted, attacked, left behind if they're being told to back up, to give disabled people space, to give your disabled child space. Start from knowing that your child doesn't need saving, your child needs empowering. There's a really big difference. We're quick to use the narrative, "I need to help this person. Or fix them. Or solve their problems. This person is a problem." It's different to say "I see the fullness of your humanity, and I'm going to empower you, to give you the tools to be who you are in the world." Recognize that you cannot *save* someone from themselves or society—but you can *empower* them.

KC: What would you say to parents who are afraid to get it wrong?
EL: You are going to make mistakes, and that's okay. You just need to evolve from it. It's better to try and get it wrong than to do nothing at all. Whether it's supporting your child, or speaking out against ableism more broadly. Learn to differentiate between trolling and constructive feedback, and take the feedback.

KC: What message do you have for parents of disabled children?
EL: It's okay to acknowledge that this is hard. It's scary when a person you love has something happen to them that can put them at risk. This person is not a tragedy, even if there is something difficult or scary. There's a lot that isn't scary about disability. There's a lot that's beautiful about it.

Chapter 2: Everything No One Tells You About Diagnosis

Experts

Dr. Brian Skotko
brianskotko.com

Dr. Emily Bronec

broadwaymedicalclinic.com/physician/emily-bronec

Lauren Clark, PhD, RN, FAAN, Professor and Shapiro Family Endowed Chair in Developmental Disability Studies at the UCLA School of Nursing

Website: www.nursing.ucla.edu/people/lauren-clark

LinkedIn: www.linkedin.com/in/lauren-clark-ba873a34

UCLAnursing on Instagram, LinkedIn, and X/Twitter

Parents

Ashequka Lacey

@babybays19 on Instagram

Jillian Hollingshead

Resources

Ages and Stages Questionnaires

agesandstages.com

American Academy of Pediatrics

www.aap.org

AAP Developmental Surveillance and Screening: www.aap.org/en/patient-care/developmental-surveillance-and-screening-patient-care

Center for Parent Information and Resources

www.parentcenterhub.org

Find Your Parent Center, by state: www.parentcenterhub.org/find-your-center

Centers for Disease Control and Prevention (CDC)

www.cdc.gov

CDC's Developmental Milestones: www.cdc.gov/ncbddd/actearly/milestones/index.html

Learn the Signs. Act Early.: www.cdc.gov/ncbddd/actearly/index.html

Undiagnosed Diseases Network
undiagnosed.hms.harvard.edu

Conversations with Experts: Dr. Brian Skotko

Dr. Brian Skotko is a board-certified medical geneticist, director of the Down Syndrome Program at Massachusetts General Hospital, and associate professor at Harvard Medical School.

KC: What would you tell families receiving a new diagnosis for their child?

BS: For every family it's a bit different, and for every child it's a bit different. I always start by saying that information should be empowering. A diagnosis can be helpful because it leads to more information. Sometimes we are not able to find that diagnosis, and it's still important to use the information that we have to embrace the person that we have, to love them, and make sure they get the maximum treatment that is available. Information can be used for good if everyone is working together, in how it's delivered, how it's processed, how it's used, and ultimately how we keep the person we love at the center of everything.

KC: Families' experiences receiving a diagnosis vary widely. Is there an ideal way to deliver a diagnosis?

BS: There really is no one way of delivering the diagnosis, but the circumstances might make a world of difference. It's important to remain human and to allow yourself to be a person talking to another person. Empathy is an important part of that process, but there are also guideposts on what to say and how and when to deliver the information. We take our lessons from the families who have been through this experience, both prenatally and postnatally.

In delivering a prenatal diagnosis, we know that parents are often in a position to make a decision about the pregnancy. What parents ask respectfully of their clinicians is to not start with a values statement: "Unfortunately, I have sad news" or "I don't know how to say this" or "I regret to have to say this" or "My heart bleeds for you." Anything that conjures up pity or sadness might not be the emotions that are felt or resonate with the parents getting the diagnosis. I oftentimes tell physicians something I've learned from the research: Just get the first line right. We know from research that the first line is remembered for a lifetime. The first sentence we recommend people saying is: "Is now a good time? Are you in a good situation to receive the news?" If it is a good time, then the recommendation from families is simply to state the results: "The results came back, suggesting that your fetus has Down syndrome (or a particular diagnosis)." It's not "I'm sorry" or "Unfortunately..." it's just the facts. And then the process of being human is the pause. The pause is so hard to practice. The silence is uncomfortable. This is the first time the couple is getting the news. They'll respond any of a number of ways and I have to sit and be there with them in a comforting silence. The couple, or the single parent, will tell us the next step. There can be questions, there can be crying, there can be denial, there can be anger. Whatever it is, take it with them from there.

In the postnatal studies, the dynamics have changed. There is no pregnancy decision on the table. We have the child in front of us. Again, to the point of being human, not starting with "I'm sorry" or "Unfortunately, I have bad news." What parents want to hear in this particular case is what all parents want to hear: "Congratulations, you've just had a baby," and point out something beautiful in that baby: the hair curls, the beautiful eyes. I have not met a baby who does not have some sparkle. Then in that conversation, and using names is very important, you say: "And I also appreciate that Elizabeth has features of Down syndrome (or other diagnosis)." And then comes the pause and following the cues of the parent.

Then, there's getting the diagnosis at nine years, ten years, forty-two years, etc. That has some special commentary as well. These are often families who have been on an exhaustive diagnostic odyssey. Getting the diagnosis in many ways is welcomed news. Finally, you have a name for it or you have a gene for it. The reaction will be quite dramatically different. But, at the same time, everyone still differs. What is most important is that the values system of the person in front of us is really the centerpiece. We need to make sure that our personal orbit as clinicians respects that and revolves around that.

KC: In your experience, both as a geneticist and a clinician, what have you learned that has surprised you?

BS: In regard to both Down syndrome and my genetics practice: The best is yet to come. Truly. Every year, when you think you've seen it all, this happens or this happens. Our genes and our medical composition do have a huge influence on our health, but something that's even a bigger influence is how societal barriers get in the way. Unfortunately and oftentimes, it can be the school system, the job market, our own families. It can be our own cultural understanding of what disability is. When those barriers are punctured and broken through, and come down, maybe even in one community, you see more potential for someone with a genetic condition. We write about these genetic conditions in our medical textbooks, but really there should be no concluding chapter, because it hasn't been written yet.

KC: What do parents need to know when they're new to parenting a disabled child?
BS: The person in front of you is the same person they were the day before you got the diagnosis. Honor that. Know that person. Allow yourself to use that diagnosis to truly try and be empowering. Parents know who their loved one is. Never let a medical professional try to define or reduce your loved one to a series of symptoms or conditions. It's the parents' role to truly know and love their child. I think that, even when things get tough and everyone is telling you no, you have to go back to "I know my child and I love them passionately." Take it one day at a time. That's enough. You've got this.

Conversations with Experts: Dr. Emily Bronec

Dr. Emily Bronec is a pediatrician whose practice focuses on compassionate, evidence-based, neurodivergent-affirming care for all children.

KC: What should I do if I suspect my child isn't developing typically?
EB: Talk to your pediatrician. Yes, you can talk to friends, but be sure to talk to your doctor always. Parents know their children best, especially with kids with disabilities or complex medical needs. You need to feel comfortable asking questions.

KC: How early can you detect disability in a child?
EB: It depends on the disability. It can be prenatally. It can happen as an infant or toddler or older.

KC: Will my pediatrician know to look out for potential disabilities or do I need to bring it up?
EB: Both. Pediatricians will do certain assessments to screen for developmental delays. However, there are many things a doctor

won't see in a fifteen-minute visit. Think about what your doctor needs to know in order to have the full picture. If you have a nagging concern, pediatricians really need to listen to that.

KC: Are all pediatricians well versed in disabilities?
EB: Every pediatrician will have done a rotation in developmental pediatrics, but that could be as little as a month. There is training, and some receive much more than others, but it varies. As a parent of a disabled child, there is a whole world that I did not know and had to learn firsthand.

KC: If my child doesn't hit all the milestones on the lists, does that mean they're disabled?
EB: Any child, even nondisabled children, can fall outside of the range of the milestones. The CDC has a list of developmental milestones that parents can use as reference. Parents can familiarize themselves with milestones as a starting point, but know that any child can vary.

KC: What sort of evaluations/screenings will my pediatrician do?
EB: If there are concerns, your doctor may ask questions about your child's development at any point. Most pediatricians will follow the American Academy of Pediatrics developmental screening guidelines. At two, four, and six months there are questions your pediatrician will ask. The formal ASQ, Ages and Stages Questionnaire, is done at nine months, eighteen months, twenty-four months, and again at age four. Typically, families fill out a questionnaire about their child's development. A developmental pediatrician or clinical psychologist will have a more detailed process.

KC: Should I be tracking things about my child that I suspect are out of the ordinary or might indicate a problem?

EB: Writing things down is really helpful. Also take videos, especially if there are movement or motor concerns. Your doctor just gets a small snapshot of your child during your visit. You can complete the picture.

KC: What if my pediatrician tells me to wait and see, and I'm not sure I feel good about that?

EB: Your pediatrician ideally should take your concerns into account. You need to feel like your pediatrician is really hearing you. You can get a second opinion. In most states, you can self-refer to Early Intervention Programs and get an evaluation and potentially access to services.

KC: What do you wish all parents knew as they begin their journey of diagnosis?

EB: It's easy to go down rabbit holes, to jump way ahead, or to catastrophize about your child's future. This gets easier with time. You get to know your child and you find hope. When you connect with other families with disabled children, your world opens up. You will meet incredible people—and your child is one of those incredible people.

Chapter 3: Everything No One Tells You About Working with Your Medical Team

Experts

Dr. Mark Borchert

www.chla.org/profile/mark-borchert-md

Dr. Gilberto Bulron

uscpediatrics.com/gastroenterology

Q'Londa Schubel

@qlonda on Instagram, TikTok, and X/Twitter

Bryan Nassour

Parents

Maya Kukes

@mayakukes on Instagram

Maya Kukes kept a blog for many years about raising a child with Down syndrome at everythingforareason-moon.blogspot.com

Resources

American Academy of Developmental Medicine and Dentistry (AADMD)

www.aadmd.org

Children's Hospital Association

www.childrenshospitals.org

Find a Children's Hospital: www.childrenshospitals.org/hospital-directory#sort=%40z95xdisplayname%20ascending

Healthcare.gov

www.healthcare.gov

Conversations with Experts: Dr. Mark Borchert

Dr. Mark Borchert is a pediatric neuro-ophthalmologist at Children's Hospital Los Angeles, where he serves as the director of the Eye Birth Defects Program and Eye Technology Program in The Vision Center. Dr. Borchert is an associate professor of clinical ophthalmology and neurology at the Keck School of Medicine of the University of Southern California.

KC: What do parents need to know as they begin this journey?
MB: You have to be willing to go on this journey *with* your child to enable them to be the best they can be. You have to be willing to abandon all your preconceived notions and expectations. Let your child help you guide them to their best. You just have to be in charge of enabling your child to get there. You are not giving up on dreams. You're giving up on preconceptions.

KC: Is it necessary for children to see pediatric specialists and not just adult doctors?
MB: Children are not little adults. Diseases that children have are distinctly different in adults. There are very few diseases that are the same in adults and children. If a doctor isn't familiar with children, the doctor can make mistakes.

KC: What should families do in advance of an appointment with their specialist?
MB: Preparing your child for the visit is the most important thing. Let them know that yes, this may seem scary, but that the doctor is here to help. Bring records from outside doctors—but don't insist that your doctor look at them. Each doctor has a different approach to evaluation, and some doctors want to evaluate patients with a clean slate. Bringing a list of questions is always a good idea. Inform the doctor up front that you have a list of questions. Parents should have expectations that their questions will be honestly answered.

KC: What makes a family difficult to work with?
MB: Parents who come in with expectations about what the doctor should say are the most challenging. If you think you know the answer, why are you coming to a doctor?

KC: If there isn't a specialist in your immediate area, is telehealth a good option?

MB: Most physicians are comfortable using telehealth for counseling, but answering questions specific to your child isn't a good idea if the physician hasn't examined the child in person first.

KC: With different conditions, do you find that the diagnosis is predictive of the outcome?

MB: It depends on the diagnosis. There are some conditions that are predictable in terms of if there will be improvement, though not always the extent of the improvement. Other conditions are not predictable at all.

KC: My doctor is talking about surgery for my child. That sounds terrifying. What do you say to parents who are afraid of surgery for their child?

MB: The best way to deal with your fear is to become educated. That's your surgeon's responsibility, to educate you on what is being done and how it can be done safely. Doctors are trained to make a judgment balancing the relative benefits and the relative risks. You can't let fear prevent you from enabling your child.

KC: Should parents limit their child's participation in activities because they are disabled?

MB: I tell parents not to hold their child back from things they want to try. They will gravitate to things they can excel at, and you won't know that in advance. If you provide them with resources, children will find a way.

*

Conversations with Experts: Dr. Gilberto Bultron

Dr. Gilberto Bultron is a pediatric gastroenterologist currently serving as director of Pediatric Gastroenterology for the Los Angeles County Department of Health Services. Dr. Bultron is chief of Pediatric Gastroenterology at LAC+USC Medical Center, director of Pediatric Gastroenterology and Pediatric Subspecialties at Olive View–UCLA Medical Center. Dr. Bultron speaks here as an individual, and not on behalf of the organizations noted here.

KC: How can parents best understand their child's symptoms and conditions?

GB: Too many parents latch on to information that they find that sounds like a cure or that sounds easy, but it may not be based in fact. Talk to your specialist. Ask questions. I know it's scary. I know you're nervous. It's okay to say: "I don't know anything about this. Here are my questions." Your doctor is here to be your partner. This is a great way to start your relationship with any doctor and to gain mutual respect.

KC: How do I know if a specialist is the right one for my child?

GB: The specialist needs to see you as an equal partner in delivering the care. Your doctor should be comfortable with you asking questions and voicing disagreement. You should feel comfortable discussing everything, especially plans of care, procedures, medications that may have side effects. Parents should never be afraid of hurting their doctor's ego by seeking a second opinion. We are all still learning about neurodivergent kids. Your specialist should also ask about you: How are you doing? What is your support network? Do you have a partner or family members who can be helpful?

KC: What is the best way for parents to track a child's symptoms?
GB: Start with writing down what is your child's baseline. What is normal for your child? Track times and days of symptoms. Be as detailed as possible. If you are tracking stools, write down the color and consistency and frequency. Many parents print out blank calendars and make notes there. If your child is able to communicate, ask your child how they are feeling and what's going on with them.

KC: How can I best prepare my child for medical experiences?
GB: Many hospitals have teaching classes. Many doctors will have the equipment in their office for teaching as well. Children will be able to learn what will happen; they will see the equipment, for example a feeding tube placed on a doll or a teddy bear. Let the child see what will happen, answer all of their questions. Let them feel like they are part of the process.

Conversations with Experts: Q'Londa Schubel

Q'Londa Schubel is a registered nurse who has worked in both home health and hospital settings.

KC: As a home care nurse, what is it like coming into a family's house for the first time?
QS: It's terrifying. I'm coming into your space and I want to be beneficial to the whole family, and I don't know if we're going to mesh well—with the patient as well as with the whole family. If you're lucky, your agency might prep you if your family has been challenging with previous nurses, but often we have little to no information.

KC: What can families do to make care a positive experience for home nurses?

QS: Be open and kind. Communication is key, even simple tips on how to soothe your child, what motivates them, or how they respond to the medical procedures you'll be performing. It's super helpful when families are organized, with their schedule, routines, expectations. I know it's hard when a stranger comes into your house to care for your child. Trust that I'm here to work together with you. We are not mind readers. We want you to tell us things. Keep in mind that we may not do things exactly as you would do them. There needs to be leeway and understanding.

KC: When we're in the hospital with our children, many of us have no experience with this, and we don't understand exactly what nurses are there to do. What exactly do nurses do?
QS: Nurses are the bridge between the patient and the doctors. We are there for twelve hours. Your doctors are not. We are drawing blood, looking at labs, running tests, and also are the doctors' eyes and ears. It's my job to relay that to the doctor. You need ice chips? I've got your ice chips. Your baby is throwing up? I'll clean that. If I can answer your questions, I will. It's not appropriate for nurses to give a specific diagnosis or results from a test. But we can get your doctor in the room to better answer those questions.

KC: Do all nurses have training working with people with disabilities?
QS: In many schools or jobs, we get the mandatory PowerPoint so they can check it off the list, but that's as deep as it goes. Technically we have been trained, but many of us haven't been exposed until we are working with disabled patients directly. Nurses appreciate when you share how we can best care for your child. We will take everything you can teach us. We want the knowledge.

KC: Parents are exhausted, grouchy, and scared when their kids are in the hospital. Is it ever okay to tell our nurses that we prefer no one comes into the room for a while?
QS: We actually prefer that. You may need alone time. You may need to sleep. Your nurse can tell you if the doctor has tests scheduled for a certain time. Sometimes the tests can be rescheduled to a different time. Whenever it's possible, we are happy adjusting our schedule to make it easier for you.

KC: How can parents be patients that the nurses want to work with?
QS: Be respectful. Be patient. Your nurse will go above and beyond for you. If you're demanding and rude and nasty, we'll still do our job, but we may not do it with a smile. Know that we are doing our best.

KC: What have you learned from your own experiences being a pediatric patient?
QS: I know firsthand what it's like to not be heard, to tell your nurses and doctors I know something is wrong, and have them dismiss me. I have had doctors look me in the eye and say, "I don't know what to do with you" because of my rare condition. I didn't know what to do either. But what I *can* do is I can ask that doctor for referrals. Ask the doctor where they would go next. Point me to the next step. Don't leave without a path forward.

KC: How can parents best empower their children with their medical team?
QS: Gather real information on your condition. Teach the child to talk to the nurses and doctors, and practice it. Your child should expect to be taken seriously. Support them in that.

Chapter 4: Everything No One Tells You About Therapies

Experts

Anna Arvisu

@aarvisu_ot on Instagram

Nikki McRory

www.mcrorypediatrics.com

@mcrory_pediatric_services on Instagram

Bryan LaScala

www.napacenter.org

www.instagram.com/napacenter

www.linkedin.com/in/bryan-lascala-76586717

Kaitlynn Hunker, MS OTR/L

Occupational therapist

Alyssa Parker VanOver, DPT

www.alyssapvanover.com

Parents

Elspeth Hetrick

Neurodivergent Parenting: Think Outside the Box: www.facebook.com/ParentingOutsideTheBoxMichigan

Resources

American Occupational Therapy Association

www.aota.org

American Physical Therapy Association

www.apta.org

American Speech-Language-Hearing Association

www.asha.org

US Department of Education: Early Intervention Program for Infants and Toddlers with Disabilities
www2.ed.gov/programs/osepeip/index.html

Conversations with Experts: Anna Arvisu

Anna Arvisu is an occupational therapist, seeing clients with a wide variety of disabilities and support needs.

KC: Will therapy "fix" my kid? Can I be guaranteed certain outcomes?
AA: We do not fix children. They're not broken. If you have an expectation of "fixing," you will be disappointed. Parents are made to feel that if their children don't get to a certain point that their children are less than. They're not. I'm not less because I'm not an NBA basketball player. We need to get rid of the "Oh, poor thing" thinking. We shouldn't pity people with different needs or skill sets. I work with children to enhance their skills, to get children to participate. I may need to adapt things or to strengthen the child's muscles. I'm not here to make your child into something that someone else needs them to be. Therapy and overall thought are shifting toward affirming neurodiversity and disability.

KC: Is therapy torture for kids?
AA: It shouldn't be. It should be client centered and play based. Children should be comfortable, even if they're doing hard things. We are always looking for the *just right challenge*. We don't want to discourage kids if it's too hard. We don't want them to be bored if it's too easy. We want them to be challenged and to feel good about it. The amount of challenge a child needs can vary from day to day. Therapists should be able to adapt for your child's

success. Your team should adapt to your child, not the other way around.

KC: How much therapy is too much? Is that a thing?
AA: That *is* a thing. Is there a lot of crying? Are they not sleeping or sleeping too much? Are they having too many days when they feel off? Are challenging behaviors increasing? Your child might be overloaded. There are times when you need to take a break. Don't let it cause an imbalance in your child's life. Play is important too.

KC: Will we have goals?
AA: We have to have goals. Funding sources need goals in order to measure progress. We set goals based on assessments. We look at what the child needs to support activities of daily living; we will set measurable and reasonable goals based on where the child is right now. Goals are reassessed often, usually every six months, and they measure the efficacy of our treatment.

KC: How can I be sure than an evaluation accurately represents my child?
AA: The therapist should do a good job of interviewing you as a parent. The therapist should really see your child from a broad, and realistic, perspective. I pride myself at looking at the big picture. I take a strength-based approach. I look at what the child can do, and how to bridge that with the things we'd like them to learn. I don't want to underestimate your child. It should be a two-way communication between parents and therapists.

KC: How much should parents be involved in the therapy sessions?
AA: That depends on the child and on the therapist. Some kids prefer not to have the parents there, and that's okay. It is my duty

as a therapist to teach parents and caregivers the skills to continue the learning at home. I'm here to help this kid learn skills that they'll generalize to everywhere they go. It's no good if the child only does the skill in the therapy setting. How do we get your child to do this at home? The more collaborative the process is with the family, the better the therapy process will be.

KC: Will my child ever graduate from therapy?
AA: Therapy shouldn't be a forever thing. Graduating from therapy looks different for everyone. It's based on making gains. We will keep going if a child continues to make gains. If your child reaches a plateau, a break might be good.

Conversations with Experts: Nikki McRory

Nikki McRory is the founder and executive director of McRory Pediatric Services, Inc.

KC: When should parents start therapies with their child?
NM: The earlier the interventions, the better the outcome. If you have a child with a known diagnosis, you can have an idea of which developmental areas are at risk. You can work on strengthening foundational skills that your child will need for later development.

KC: Do you find that a child's diagnosis is predictive of their outcomes?
NM: There's a common saying: "If you've seen one child with autism, you've seen *one* child with autism." This applies to all disabilities. You cannot generalize too much. You will always see a large range of strengths and challenges. Every child is capable of learning and of making progress.

KC: If a pediatrician isn't concerned but a parent is, is it appropriate for a parent to seek interventions on their own?
NM: Trust your gut. It's always okay to seek an evaluation. You may have your suspicions validated, or you may learn you're wrong, and that's okay too. You'll never regret having your child assessed and gaining the knowledge either way.

KC: This guy online says that he can help my child. He has a fancy therapy he developed himself. He even certified himself in it! Ooh, and he sells supplements! And they're on sale!
NM: Make sure you are going to licensed professionals. Make sure they are using evidence-based interventions. Ask questions. What are the risks? Is this worth those risks? Will any treatment or supplement counteract other medications your child has been prescribed? You need to talk to your doctor about everything to make sure it will be safe for your child.

KC: How can parents best support their child's development outside of therapy sessions?
NM: Maximize opportunities for learning. But always be a parent first. Parents don't need to be therapists all day with their child. Work lessons into your daily routines. Think about the things you're already doing with your child: taking a bath, having a snack, getting dressed. Each of these things is an opportunity for learning. Don't feel guilty if you're not turning every moment into a therapy session. That shouldn't be the expectation. If everything becomes therapy, it's too much and it's not sustainable, or even fun, for anyone.

KC: Can therapy be fun for children?
NM: Therapy should be a fun process for children. It should feel like play, especially in early intervention. When children play with

others, they're working on joint attention, engagement, attachment, bonding. They're exploring their world, working on motor skills, learning sensory information. When they're sitting or on their tummy, they're developing muscles that they'll need for crawling and walking. They're working on hand-eye coordination every time they put a puzzle or a shape sorter together. The Fred Rogers quote about play is spot on: "Play is often talked about as if it were a relief from serious learning. But for children play IS serious learning. Play is really the work of childhood."

Conversations with Experts: Bryan LaScala

Bryan LaScala is the chief executive officer of the NAPA Center.

KC: What can parents do to prepare their children for a positive therapy experience?

BL: Talk to your child in advance about the experience. Regardless of your child's level of communication, you can show them pictures of the space, show them videos, talk with them about what will happen.

KC: What is the NAPA Center and why is it unique?

BL: We specialize in intensive therapy programs, all are in three-week increments, and each session varies depending on the program for the child. For families considering intensive therapy, find a provider who has done intensive therapy before. Trust that person to provide a recommendation for your child, and then let your child show you what they can do. We never want to overprescribe therapy. Our long-term goal is to bring every child to their full developmental potential. We work toward the wins along the way to arrive at what full potential looks like for each child. Focusing on head control can be a huge win. Don't miss those celebratory moments.

KC: How can parents best support their children after intensive therapy sessions or outside of their regularly scheduled therapy?
BL: Be realistic. Ask your therapist what are the best things you can do with your child, and let them know how much time you realistically have to dedicate to therapy at home. It can be tough to be a parent and also to be your child's therapist at home.

KC: How can parents best communicate with and support therapists working with their child?
BL: Communicate your child's needs, likes, dislikes, and motivations, especially at the beginning. Also, think about what support you need as a parent in order to trust your therapy team. There is a lot of trust and communication that needs to happen in order to best support your child.

Chapter 5: Everything No One Tells You About Insurance and Government Benefits

Experts

Mary Foley
Medicaid, Medicare CHIP Dental Services Association (MDSA): www.medicaiddental.org/about

Leslie Lobel
undivided.io
@undividedapp on Instagram
www.linkedin.com/company/teamundivided

Abbi Coursolle
National Health Law Program: healthlaw.org/team/abbi-coursolle

Judy Mark
Disability Voices United: disabilityvoicesunited.org

Parents

Effie Parks
effieparks.com
Once Upon a Gene podcast: effieparks.com/podcast

Resources

Administration for Community Living (ACL)
acl.gov
ACL Support for Caregivers: acl.gov/programs/support-caregivers

Centers for Medicaid and Medicare Services
www.cms.gov

Children's Health Insurance Program (CHIP)
www.medicaid.gov/chip/index.html

US Department of Education: Early Intervention Program
www2.ed.gov/programs/osepeip/index.html

HealthCare.gov Glossary
www.healthcare.gov/glossary

Medicaid
www.medicaid.gov
State Overviews: www.medicaid.gov/state-overviews/index.html
Medicaid and CHIP Eligibility and Enrollment Webinars: www.medicaid.gov/resources-for-states/medicaid-and-chip-eligibility-enrollment-webinars/index.html

Conversations with Experts: Mary Foley

Mary Foley is the executive director of the Medicaid, Medicare CHIP Services Dental Association (MDSA).

KC: If my child is disabled, does that mean they will automatically qualify for government benefits?

MF: It depends on the state and the disability. The word "disability" is very broad. It is interpreted in different ways by the federal government and by state governments. The eligibility criteria for your state determines if your child qualifies for benefits. The key thing the parent will want to do is to understand: How does the state define disability? What disabilities are included in the eligibility criteria? You don't get benefits unless you're eligible under your state's criteria. You can search online: "Medicaid benefits eligibility Indiana." Search for your specific state, and also look at www.medicaid.gov for federal guidelines.

KC: How can I find out what services exist in my state and what providers take Medicaid?

MF: Medical providers or social service systems should be able to provide contact information for your state's Medicaid agency. Calling your local children's hospital can be a good place to start, especially if you are able to speak with their social worker.

KC: Are government health insurance benefits income based?

MF: Medicaid first looks at family income for eligibility. If your income falls at or below the state level, you are probably eligible, regardless of disability. If your family is not eligible under the income criteria, the second way to potentially qualify is by disability.

KC: I've heard of CHIP—what is that?

MF: CHIP is the Children's Health Insurance Program, established in the 1990s. It covers healthcare services for children whose families have a low income, but whose income is above that needed to qualify for Medicaid. The CHIP program often covers healthcare services for children from families who do not have an employer-based healthcare plan.

KC: Do CHIP and Medicaid cover different things?
MF: Both CHIP and Medicaid include a mandate for dental coverage as well as medical. CHIP is not mandated under federal law to provide all medically necessary services. Medicaid is obligated to cover all medically necessary services. With CHIP there can be an annual or lifetime cap, or other limitations of services. Medicaid does have limitations, but if the services are medically necessary, then they may be approved. Both CHIP and Medicaid rules are set by each individual state, and these may vary from state to state. Some states combine their CHIP and Medicaid programs. If combined, the broader benefit would be covered for the child.

KC: Okay, so I'm sitting down to do the paperwork. It's a lot. Like, really a lot.
MF: It's like a college application. Take a deep breath. There are no quick answers. It's a process. You have to submit lots of documentation to demonstrate that your child is really eligible. There will be renewal paperwork every year, though that will be less than the initial application.

KC: I'm reading all of this and my eyes are glazing over and I feel like I don't understand it. Is it just me? Is there some secret way to figure it all out?
MF: Healthcare delivery and insurance programs can be incredibly difficult. Everyone experiences challenges signing up and trying to get coverage. There are many forms to sort through and a lot of unfamiliar terms to understand. It's hard for everyone, and families with language barriers have even more challenges.

KC: What do you wish families know when they're starting this process?

MF: As soon as your child is diagnosed, start on a path of self-education. Learn about the program rules in your state. Go slow. It will take time. Often, families don't seek services until they are urgent or their child is in pain. And then, they often get frustrated because the process is taking so long. Families should prioritize preventative care, going regularly for well medical and dental checkups. For children with complex medical conditions, preventative dental care often isn't a priority, because other conditions take precedence. However, by not going for routine preventative services, problems can emerge, and soon an emergency exists. Prepare now. Schedule your dental appointments early and regularly, and make sure that you have all of your insurance paperwork updated and in place.

Conversations with Experts: Leslie Lobel

Leslie Lobel is the director of Health Plan Advocacy for Undivided, a platform for supporting families raising children with disabilities and developmental delays.

KC: Why is this all so overwhelming? Is it all really that hard?

LL: The system is not set up to be user-friendly. The way to make it easier on yourself: know what your plan knows from the start. Find out what your plan covers.

KC: Why does it matter if I know the specifics of my child's insurance coverage?

LL: Our families cannot afford to not know what the benefits and coverage are. Our families need to know if OT, PT, speech, behavioral interventions, and mental health services are covered. We need to understand if services have limits and what those are. We need to understand if we'll get the same reimbursement in January that we'll get in December. Figure out at what point during the year you'll get reimbursed for your deductible. You may get no reimbursement for the beginning of the year, since everything will be processing to your deductible. But, by the end of the year, you could be seeing a good percentage of what you have paid. You can really begin to budget.

KC: How will knowing this information help me in planning my child's care?

LL: Once you have this information, families can plan and make the best decisions they can based on the insurance they have. They can plan for the current year, and can plan in an ongoing way. They can balance those benefits with other funding sources, can make an overall treatment plan, can decide what to ask insurance or school for. First, you need to understand what each system provides. Then, you can make the best choices.

KC: What am I not thinking of in terms of what I need to know about my plan?

LL: Audit your plan every year: Figure out what's going on and if there are any changes from the previous year. Do not assume that your plan year is the calendar year. Know when your plan year renews. This helps you figure out what you will be liable for in- and out-of-network deductibles. It can help you figure out where in the year to buy a big-ticket item via insurance, such as medical equipment. Ask if this is a separate deductible or part of your main deductible. The plan is always going to be stacked against you. The more you know, the more you can try and even the playing field in your favor. It's not set up to be advantageous to you. They're not your friends. Be an informed participant. Know where to push and where to back away. Know what the plan is obligated to do.

KC: This takes forever. I'm so sick of hold music. How do I make these phone calls as quick and painless as possible?
LL: Don't call under a time crunch. Give yourself time. Avoid calling on Mondays or on the first of the month. Try calling early in the morning or in the evening. Ask the representative what are the least busy times to call, and what their customer service hours are. Have work to do in the background for when you're on hold. Clean up your inbox, fold laundry, tidy your desktop, play online mahjong. Make the wait time valuable to you so you're not resentful of the time spent.

KC: I finally got a human on the phone. And they're totally unhelpful. What now?
LL: Don't be afraid to ask for a supervisor if you aren't getting the answers you need. If the person you're speaking with can't do it, that doesn't mean it can't be done. Some people are problem solvers and some are problem makers. Find the helpful, curious people. The best people are the ones who are interested in you as a person. If you're on the phone with someone who isn't helpful or well trained, you can end the call and call back and speak with someone else.

KC: It's all their fault. They're terrible.
LL: Maybe. But you are part of this team. Don't just hold your plan accountable. Hold yourself accountable. Start a spreadsheet. My big advice to people: Start a claims spreadsheet for out-of-network claims. Audit your plan. Determine if it's worthwhile to submit out-of-network claims. If you don't keep the spreadsheet, you can't assume that you remembered to file every single claim. A fully processed year of claims is a failure for the plan and a success

for you. You may forget to submit February, but your spreadsheet won't forget. Your spreadsheet will always remember.

KC: Oh. So, does that mean I should open this giant stack of letters from my insurance plan?
LL: Those are likely your Explanation of Benefits (EOBs). The mail is scary. I get it. But it contains information you need. Every claim generates an EOB. It's the story of every claim and of every medical experience. It shows you if you are getting reimbursed, or if money went toward your deductible. If it was denied, there will be a denial code, and the code will be explained on that page. If you need to call the plan about a claim, you should have this in front of you so you can explain the problem to them. There will also be information on how to file a grievance or an appeal. It's important information for you to understand.

KC: I can't figure out if certain things are covered. What about things like diapers or wheelchairs or adaptive equipment?
LL: After you've read your plan's Summary of Benefits and Coverage (SBC), you can call to ask your plan for things that you're not clear on. It's always better to call after you have done your detective work. For things like diapers, wheelchairs, equipment, etc. those might be covered under a category called durable medical equipment (DME) or expendables. Call your plan and ask if there is a DME benefit. Ask for their terminology. Diapers may be called incontinence supplies, and that category may also cover things like disposable pads, diapers liners, waterproof mattress covers, incontinence spray. If you want to access your DME benefit, you'll need a prescription from the doctor that lists all the items, the size, and the quantity per month. Ask your plan if there are quantity limits per month. Your plan can also give you a list of

in-network providers, or ask your doctor's office if they have suppliers. If a DME company is in-network, they can often help you navigate your insurance plan. Be sure to ask your plan if there's a separate deductible for DME, or if there's an annual limit. This can help you plan when it is best to order these items.

KC: There's a thing that's not covered. I'm trying to get it covered by another source. They're saying I need a denial letter. What is that and how do I get one?
LL: This can also be called a letter of noncoverage. Knowing the right terminology can unlock what you need. Ask them. It can be tricky to get a letter. But it may be necessary to get it covered elsewhere. If you have an employer plan, you can call your human resources department. You can call your insurance plan, and you may need to speak with a supervisor. Make it clear that you're not trying to get the service covered, you're just proving that it is not covered by your plan. If they won't send an actual letter, have them send you the exact text in their literature that explains what is and is not covered.

KC: I think I need to file an appeal. How do I make it successful?
LL: The essential thing about appeals is understanding the difference between "I need" and "I want." The plan is not interested in "I want." You can't talk about what you want. You MUST talk about what the plan **needs** to do. You need to prove that your child is being denied access to medically necessary services. The plan needs to provide you with **access to care**. It's not just "I want this provider rather than that provider." That's what out-of-network benefits are for. It's "I need to be able to have access to care; no one in network can provide this service, so you need to provide me access. Here is the doctor's letter and prescription proving that it is

medically necessary." Only argue for things that are covered benefits. You need to understand what your plan actually covers. And everything must be supported by a doctor as medically necessary.

KC: That sounds like a lot of work.

LL: It is. In addition to gathering the supporting paperwork, you may need to call every provider in network to show that the plan does not cover anyone who can provide the medically necessary services to your child. Be specific. "No one in network has experience with my child's diagnosis. My child needs feeding therapy and no in-network providers offer that. Your providers only offer thirty-minute therapy sessions and my child cannot make progress without sixty-minute sessions." Everything needs to support your doctor's letter of medical necessity. Do not make any statements you are not sure of. Tell a compelling story based on facts. Address every reason that the plan has denied a claim. If they give you four reasons for denial, address all four. It's easy for them to deny again if you don't answer everything.

KC: This is all really stressful.

LL: You'll incur short-term stress learning about your plan, but in the long term you'll reduce stress. Once it's in place, it saves you time and money. You may never love dealing with your health plan, but your child needs you to be effective. In my life, I had no control over the upheaval in our lives with our child. I found that insurance is a place where I could have some control. I could make sure that my child got full use of this plan. It got her the care that got her the best outcome. When you win, it's great.

Chapter 6: Everything No One Tells You About Individualized Education Programs (IEPs)

Experts

Lisa Mosko Barros

SpEducational: www.speducational.org

Valerie Vanaman

Vanaman German, LLP: www.vanamangerman.com

Markeisha Hall

www.markeishahall.com

Parents

Erick Puell, MA, NBCT

Public elementary school inclusion instructional coach

Resources

Center for Parent Information and Resources

www.parentcenterhub.org

Council of Parent Attorneys and Advocates, Inc.

www.copaa.org

Glossary of Education Reform

www.edglossary.org

Individuals with Disabilities Education Act (IDEA)

sites.ed.gov/idea

Parents and Families: sites.ed.gov/idea/parents-families

US Department of Education

A Guide to the Individualized Education Program: www2.ed.gov/parents/needs/speced/iepguide/index.html

Wrightslaw

www.wrightslaw.com

*

Conversations with Experts: Valerie Vanaman

Valerie Vanaman is a special education attorney and managing partner of Vanaman German, LLP.

KC: What do you wish every parent knew about the IEP process?
VV: Prior to 1974, there was no special education. The US Constitution does not include a right to education. It was all created by statute. People don't realize the work that went into getting where we've gotten, and what it looks like without it. Our grandparents knew what it was like to not have it. It's not perfect, no matter how skilled your lawyer is.

KC: Do families need a lawyer for their child's IEP?
VV: It's highly individualized. If it's contentious, it's best to have a lawyer. For districts offering alternate dispute resolution, be wary of the district attempting to offer the bare minimum, which would not truly address the child's needs. If it's clear that services are not being delivered, that certain kinds of communication are not being allowed, or other scenarios, a lawyer is necessary.

KC: When should families meet with a lawyer?
VV: If families have the resources and time, they should meet with a lawyer before the IEP. If there are no issues with the IEP, then families who have not met with a lawyer prior to the IEP do not need to see a lawyer. If there are issues or if it is contentious, meet with a lawyer at the first signs of concern.

KC: How do I know if I have the right lawyer?
VV: You need to make sure you have professionals who will be straight with you, and not sugarcoat anything. You need to be

willing to make it clear that you want the hard answers—you do yourself a disservice by not hearing both the best *and* the worst.

KC: Who are the best clients to work with?
VV: Serious clients who are looking for good advice, and are open to hearing the realm of possibility. Families who do best are open-minded enough to seek the range of options, and to question why they want what they are asking for for their child. They have done research but are open to discussion.

KC: What should families bring to their first meeting with a lawyer?
VV: Bring a timeline. I can't emphasize that enough. Include date of diagnosis, doctor visits and notes, school chronology, etc. It's much easier to update a timeline than to try and remember dates when you are meeting with your lawyer, or to go back and attempt to re-create a timeline. Bring key documents such as diagnostic reports and any academic documents—teacher reports, prior IEPs, etc.

KC: Are families generally happy with the outcome of their IEP process?
VV: That's different for each family. The goal is to achieve an acceptable outcome that delivers FAPE for your child. Families have a difficult time when they believe that their child is legally entitled to what is *best.* There is no law that says your child is entitled to what is *best.* Only what is *meaningful.*

KC: Does the IEP process get easier?
VV: There are years of grace and years of turmoil. I don't think any family has gone through it without bumps. I can go several years without seeing a family, then they need to come in again.

There are stable periods, periods of adjustment, learning curves, and changes along the way.

Conversations with Experts: Markeisha Hall

Markeisha Hall is a special education advocate and IEP coach.

KC: What would you tell parents starting on their IEP journey?
MH: Think about how your kids can access everything in the whole school day. This isn't just about academics. It's about your child as a whole person. Your child's worth isn't in their grades. Recess, field trips, library time. Whatever they enjoy, it matters. Think about your vision for your child and celebrate their strengths. The IEP prepares your child for independence, future education, or employment.

KC: Parents are equal partners in the IEP process. What does this mean? How can parents genuinely be equal partners if they're coming in not knowing how to do this?
MH: It's as simple as it sounds: your voice and what you have to contribute has weight, just as much as everyone else's voice. You can add ideas and goals even if you don't have the right terminology. The best way to be an equal member is to have all the information they have. Every time before the meeting, you need a draft of the IEP. Highlight what you don't understand. Write questions on it. Give yourself time. You can talk to your team, get clarification, ask questions in advance of the IEP meeting. You can't make decisions in advance of the meeting, but you can always ask questions. The more you understand, the more you can participate.

KC: What do families of color need to know about how their children might be treated differently?

MH: The statistics are there. This happens. Know what your rights are. Know what assessments can and can't be done. Be prepared to talk about behavior. There is overdiagnosis of behaviors with African American students, and this puts children disproportionately into special education. You can decline special education if you don't believe that is the appropriate placement. You know your child.

KC: What should parents know about IEP goals?

MH: Consider looking at your goals in terms of your vision for your child's future—not just a year from now, but as they become adults. What will most benefit your child to become their best future self? What does my child need to start working on now to gain maximum independence? How can we build goals from my child's strengths, not just from deficits? Create a vision statement and build goals that will get your child there.

KC: What's a vision statement and how does it work with my child's IEP?

MH: As parents, we are working for the best version of life for all of our children, disabled or not. Your child is more than just what is in an IEP document. Create a vision statement of where you see them when they become adults. Build it around their strengths, what they love, and how they can achieve maximum independence and autonomy. Include your child in creating the vision statement. The statement can evolve as your child gets older. And it can inform how you create goals for an IEP and where you focus your child's time.

Chapter 7: Everything No One Tells You About School

Experts

Julissa Zamudio
Public school elementary special education teacher

Dina Marie Swann
Public school elementary and middle school inclusion facilitator and teacher

Parents

Rachel Ulriksen
thekevinchronicles.com

Kristen Gray
The Gray Academy: thegrayacademy.org

Resources

Canva: Visual Suite for Everyone
www.canva.com

***Our Three Little Birds*: profile template for schools using Canva**
our3lilbirds.blogspot.com/2017/05/how-to-make-one-page-profile-ellie-style.html

Disability Rights Education and Defense Fund (DREDF): Parent Training and Information Center
dredf.org/special-education/parent-training-and-information-center/

Conversations with Experts: Julissa Zamudio

Julissa Zamudio is an elementary school special education teacher.

KC: What should parents tell teachers about their student at the beginning of a school year?

JZ: A teacher gets so many IEPs at once. It's so much easier if on the first day parents let you know what their child needs. It's great if parents can write down one page or make a list.

KC: How often should parents be in communication with their child's teacher?

JZ: Ideally, always have open communication. Ask your teacher their preferred way to communicate: emails, texts, phone calls, or in person. I see more growth with kids whose parents communicate with me, because I learn what I need to know to teach their child better.

KC: What would you say to parents who are afraid to send children with disabilities to school?

JZ: This happens a lot, especially when kids are going from preschool to kindergarten. It breaks my heart when parents come to me and ask, "Should my child even be in school?" Yes. Your child deserves the same experience as everyone else. Be honest with your child's teacher about your concerns and feelings. What does your child need for safety or comfort? Do we need to create breaks for medication? How do we motivate your child? What do they love? Develop a plan together. If your child is starting a new school, take a walk or drive past the school, practice the morning routine. When their child is in school, parents can come to the classroom to observe.

KC: Have you had to work with families on accepting their child's disability?

JZ: Too often, I see when families feel broken. No one has explained to them that it's okay. Parents are asking me, "Will my child be okay?" Yes. Yes, they will be okay. They may have different milestones. That is okay. Your child is on their time, not on our time. Have high expectations for your child. But also be flexible. Meet them where they are. Believe your child is capable.

KC: Have you seen different cultures playing into a family's view of their child's disability?
JZ: Very much so. Teachers always need to take a student's culture into account. I find I have to break stereotypes of disability. I encourage the family to ask questions, to talk about it if they're coming from a culture where they feel they're supposed to hide their disabled child. This is something teachers see, and they can both respect the family's culture and show families all the ways that their child is amazing. In some families, regardless of culture, parents focus on what kids can't do so much that they don't see all the things their child *can* do.

KC: What would you say to families who don't speak the same primary language as the teacher?
JZ: Ask for a translator. Use apps that you can set to your language. I use apps for parent communication that parents can set to their own language. It may be easier for parents to text or email so they can put your response into a translation app. Teachers and parents need to take the time to find ways to communicate. Don't give up. Come to the meetings. We want you there.

KC: How often do your students surprise you with how well they do in school?
JZ: Every. Single. Day. Focus on what they can do and they will amaze you every day.

*

Conversations with Experts: Dina Marie Swann

Dina Marie Swann is an elementary and middle school inclusion facilitator.

KC: Should my child be in special education, general education, or split their days between the two?

DMS: It depends on the child. Your child *is* capable. Use the least restrictive environment (LRE) model: Ask yourself if the appropriate supports can be provided in a general education setting. As a parent, prioritize your child, how they learn best, and what their optimum future looks like. Look at what can best serve your child and their future plan.

KC: What would you say to parents who are nervous about placing their child in a more inclusive setting?

DMS: Ask how you can ensure your child is getting everything they need to meet their physical and medical needs, as well as their academic and social needs. I advise parents to think about their child ten years from now. What will their life look like? What sort of program will they be in? Will they have aged out of the school system? What is the optimum vision of your child's future? School inclusion creates a realistic opportunity to participate in the community, to be able to functionally communicate, to deal with environmental concerns. What opportunities does your child need now to prepare them for this future?

KC: Students of color are disproportionately placed into more restrictive environments. What do parents of students of color

need to know in order to make sure their children are on the most appropriate path for them?
DMS: Historically, this happens over and over. A strong teacher or administrator will have the ability to recognize their own bias, and will be willing to address that in order to objectively look at the child's learning style and what the child needs. Ask if your school or your school district has committees dedicated to disproportionality and Black student success.

KC: Are there disadvantages to being in an inclusive setting?
DMS: Parents of children in full inclusion may need to seek information, because it may not be built into conversations in the same way. At a special education school, all the children are preparing for their transitions into adulthood, and that information is automatically provided to families. Without that being built in, your job as a parent is to seek out the information.

KC: Are all teachers trained in special education?
DMS: Every teacher should be trained in special education. But that's not always the reality. We need to support a bridge between special education and general education. Every child is individual. Ideally, we should all be able to individualize. It's hard with a large class size. We need to recognize neurodivergence, and how to meet children where they are. If your school doesn't have an inclusion facilitator, ask your teacher how they will modify schoolwork and projects so that your child can access them. Parents can be proactive for their children. Parents and teachers can always find ways to celebrate their children together.

KC: Do you find that parents have a clear idea of how their child's IEP is being followed?

DMS: Not at all. The biggest advice I can give to parents is to ask teachers and service providers for an update on a regular basis. Sometimes it naturally happens. Having a relationship with parents contributes hugely to my success. If parents ask for an email at least monthly from service providers and teachers, it holds them accountable. Providers know that they'll be getting an email from parents, so it keeps your child top of mind. If providers share information on what would be beneficial to do with the child at home, the parents can be accountable for that, and learning can translate at home as well.

KC: Do I need to do all the school things at home in order for my child to be successful?
DMS: Providers need to be realistic and have empathy for the family. Reinforcement at home is ideal, but we understand that you have multiple kids or you need to make dinner or take a shower. It can be unrealistic to expect a child to do too many things at home. We need to work together with families to create a plan. Time with family is precious. This alone can support everything they are doing at school. Always keep in mind your child's optimum future. Work from there. Is your child's priority to pass physics or is it to live independently? What can they learn now that will achieve that? What is the future you are fighting for?

KC: What do I do if my child isn't yet able to communicate what their vision is for their optimum future and I just don't know what it looks like?
DMS: A teacher's job is to talk about that with you, to help you plan for that future. An optimum future can happen with an AAC [Augmentative and Alternative Communication] device or a trach or whatever accommodations your child needs to be their best. What

exposure does your child need to general education to make that happen? What is your family structure like? Do you want your child going out into the community more? How can I introduce that at a school level? How do we build rich experiences for your child? We need to think about what is important for your child to learn.

KC: I don't know if my child will ever be fully independent. Do we really need to be thinking about independence now?
DMS: All kids are working on skills that bring them toward independence, not just disabled kids. You want optimum success for any kid. You need to teach them more than just to rely on you, even in small ways. You need to think about what independence looks like for them, how they live the best version of their future. It starts in school.

Chapter 8: Everything No One Tells You About Disability Rights and Advocacy

Experts

Maria Town
American Association of People with Disabilities (AAPD): www.aapd.com
@maria_town on Instagram
cpshoes.tumblr.com

Elena Hung
Little Lobbyists: littlelobbyists.org

Parents

AnGèle Cade
A Kid Like Aundon: www.akidlikeaundon.org

Resources

Americans with Disabilities Act (ADA)
www.ada.gov

ADA National Network
adata.org

Disabled Parenting Project
disabledparenting.com

Crip Camp **documentary**
cripcamp.com

Ki'tay Davidson
obamawhitehouse.archives.gov/blog/2013/08/15/championing-our-communities-open-letter

National Disability Rights Network (NDRN)
www.ndrn.org
NDRN Member Agencies (select by state): www.ndrn.org/about/ndrn-member-agencies

Inclusion International
inclusion-international.org

American Academy of Developmental Medicine and Dentistry (AADMD)
www.aadmd.org
AADMD Toolkits: www.aadmd.org/toolkits

Conversations with Experts: Maria Town

Maria Town is the president and CEO of the American Association of People with Disabilities (AAPD) and is the former senior associate director of the White House Office of Public Engagement during the Obama administration.

KC: What is the American Association of People with Disabilities (AAPD)?
MT: The AAPD is a national cross-disabilities civil rights organization that works to increase the economic and political power of the more than sixty million disabled people across the United States. We are disability-led and focus on disabled people being leaders in communities and organizations.

KC: How does the AAPD define disability?
MT: We cite the definition in the ADA. Any mental or physical impairment that impacts an activity of daily living. That definition is intentionally very broad. The ADA was designed to provide rights and protections for as many people as possible. There is no hierarchy of disability, or judgment of who is "disabled enough."

KC: Why is it so essential for disabled people to be in front of disability advocacy, and not just a bunch of well-meaning parents?
MT: For way too long, people with disabilities have been denied opportunities to speak for ourselves. We are the experts in our own experience. Parents also have a lot of expertise. In my own life, I've seen that the person who sees my limitations the most is my mother. This isn't a bad thing. It's because she has had to worry about what my disability will mean for me from the start. She has had to fight for my inclusion. She was so supportive of me. This allowed me not to see what all those stakes were. She has never stopped seeing those stakes. It can be hard for parents to give their children the space to take risks. I don't know if any parent is able to fully let go. That impacts how they engage in advocacy. Parents put children into many therapies, all to develop their voice. But too often, when we raise our voice, we're told to be quiet.

As a parent, can you separate the stakes from your child's experience? As disabled people, we see the stakes, but we see them differently.

KC: We know that it's important for our disabled children to see disabled role models. Why is it important for everyone, regardless of their abilities, to see disabled role models?
MT: Representation matters. Growing up, I did not see another woman with cerebral palsy who had a career until I was twenty-three. Having disabled mentors opens up what we view as possible. It gives us a clearer picture of what our future can look like. Part of what reinforces stigma is the absence of authentic representation. There's a fervent belief that disability is not only bad but specifically undesirable, that it is this exceptional thing that happens that you don't want. But disability is a natural part of the human condition. Most of us will become disabled eventually. But society and institutions have had the privilege of pretending like disability doesn't exist.

KC: It is harder to be disabled than not to be disabled. So many parents feel ashamed to say "This is hard." What would you say to those parents?
MT: You need to say it. Disability isn't bad. But it is hard. There are times when I have to recognize what I can and cannot do in a way my nondisabled peers don't have to. Saying this is hard is way more empowering than trying to grin and bear it. Parents need to acknowledge that this is hard—the systems make this hard. You'll be required to jump through hoops to get your child what they need. Parents need to say it's hard so that their children have the skills to realize that the problem is not *them* but is the systems they are confronting.

KC: Can I prevent my child from having internalized ableism?
MT: Internalized ableism is a beast. Even the most proud disabled person deals with it. What I would hope that parents and family members can realize is that their goal should not only be access and inclusion for their loved one but also making sure their child grows up with as little internalized ableism as possible. It's a tough thing to do if your child has to go through all these therapies in order to achieve. The message they can get is that they need to be as nondisabled as possible, or that they need to pass. That is a really damaging message, because one day they will realize that they can't do it anymore, and they will not have the skills to manage that realization. The goal should never be to make your child compliant. Instead, we need to ask ourselves, "How do we create environments for our kids to thrive?" We need to create spaces where everyone belongs as they are.

Conversations with Experts: Elena Hung

Elena Hung is the cofounder of the kid-centered disability advocacy group Little Lobbyists.

KC: What was your path to creating Little Lobbyists?
EH: I started the organization, back in 2017 with the Affordable Care Act (ACA) repeal efforts in the news. My friends and I got really worried. And scared. And angry. The narrative in the media did not talk about families like ours. There was a sense of urgency. I talked to everybody who would talk to me. We learned from disabled adults and activists. We sought out disabled leaders, and asked them what their experience was like as a child. They know how to combine the personal story with the advocacy. That was the key to our organization.

KC: Little Lobbyists actively involves and centers the kids. Why is this so important?

EH: This IS about the kids, so of course they should be front and center. I was very well aware of how disabled children have been portrayed and used in terms of media and previous advocacy efforts. We talk a lot about Jerry's Kids and parading children to raise money, and you see this in other organizations too. It evokes pity; people express pity via their donations. That was on our minds from early on. We wanted to put a face on the issue—by telling real stories rather than evoking pity. My daughter is joyful and happy. We wanted people to see children who are visibly disabled and also having fun as children. A kid can have a ventilator and still be out at the playground having fun. What I would have given as a NICU mom to have seen this picture: a child like mine, hooked up to a ventilator, on a swing, happy at a playground. From the first day we were on Capitol Hill, we were showing who was being directly impacted: the patient. It shouldn't be revolutionary to center our kids, but it has been. This is not charity. This is community. We fight for all kids, not just our own: collective liberation, collective change.

KC: How exactly does telling our children's stories change the narrative?

EH: We are literally putting a face on the policy or issue. We focus on how we present our children, and the narrative we want to tell. We ask families to write about their child's personality, not just a list of symptoms. Everything we do humanizes our children, on social media, in advocacy, everywhere. "She's three and she loves *Sesame Street*" gives you a connection in a way that starting off naming a rare disease doesn't. We tell the story of our child, or they tell it themselves, and then we explain how a certain policy would impact our family. Always tie a personal story to the advocacy.

KC: Do you just call a senator and ask for a meeting?
EH: That's how it's supposed to work. Sometimes we set meetings. Sometimes we just show up, always with our disabled kids. If you as an elected official don't have time to meet with your constituents, your constituents will find someone who does.

KC: What would you say to parents who fear their children would be disruptive in meetings?
EH: It starts with the child's safety and with their comfort level. We have had to adapt to make it work for them. We encourage our kids to speak, with words or signs or an AAC device. Everyone has a seat at the table. For our kids, that can be in a chair or sitting on the table or walking around the room or laying down. When we feed our kids with feeding tubes, that normalizes it for people who have never seen that before. It's very different than just a parent coming in and talking about their child who is tube fed. We're educating staffers by just living our lives.

KC: What do you wish your representatives understood?
EH: Normalizing the care experience: what independence means, what interdependence means, and where disabled children belong in the community. Not long ago, a child like mine would have been institutionalized. We need Home- and Community-Based Services (HCBS) so we can get services without institutionalization. It's not our child's disability that is the problem; it's the lack of support, the lack of services, the constant fight—*that* is the trauma. If we make care part of every policy, disabled children will really be part of the community, as they're meant to be, and they'll grow up to be adults who are part of the community, as they're meant to be.

KC: If parents want to get involved in advocacy, what do you suggest they do?
EH: You don't have to come to Washington, DC, to make a change. Get to know your local representatives. Get involved in your local elections. It does matter who gets voted into office. It determines who will have meetings with you. If we have more disabled people in office, they would have a different understanding of these issues. Make advocacy part of your life. At the grocery store, if someone is staring at your kid, that's an opportunity for advocacy.

KC: What has advocacy taught you that you've taken into your organization?
EH: You can advocate for your kid, and you can also advocate for all kids. Community building translates into the storytelling and the representation that we're doing: Disabled kids are kids, are having fun, are fully human, just like other kids. We're teaching our children that there's a place for them. We talk about survive and thrive—for the parents as well as the kids. If we're doing one and not the other, we're missing the point of this. We have to find joy. We have to create joy when we can't find it. It's important for my children to see me joyful. It's important for them to see the hope.

Chapter 9: Everything No One Tells You About Financial Planning and Future Care Plans

Experts

Mark Solomon
snfguidance.com

Josh Fishkind
Hope Trust: hopetrust.com

Shawn Francis

agents.worldfinancialgroup.com/shawn-francis

Just Two Dads podcast: www.facebook.com/wearejusttwodads/

theamazingxperience.wordpress.com

Tamra Pauly

Person Centered Projects: personcenteredprojects.com

Parents

Ellen Ladau

disabledparenting.com/author/ellen-ladau/

Resources

National Association of Councils on Developmental Disabilities

nacdd.org

Special Needs Answers (find a special needs planner)

specialneedsanswers.com

Administration for Community Living (ACL)

acl.gov

ACL Person-centered planning (PCP): acl.gov/programs/consumer-control/person-centered-planning

The Arc

thearc.org

National Disability Institute (NDI)

www.nationaldisabilityinstitute.org

NDI financial planning template: www.nationaldisabilityinstitute.org/wp-content/uploads/2021/04/star-goal-setting-worksheet-ndi-tool.pdf

National Guardianship Association (NGA)

www.guardianship.org

Special Needs Alliance (SNA)
www.specialneedsalliance.org

Conversations with Experts: Mark Solomon

Mark Solomon is a financial guidance specialist for families of disabled children, with a focus on helping families achieve financial security for both now and the future.

KC: What does a special needs financial planner do?
MS: Expenses are even tighter for families of disabled children. People use money and time as their excuse for not being proactive in their planning. But you can't help anyone, and especially not your child, if you don't have a clear sense of your finances. I provide financial guidance for families of disabled children, based on their idea of financial security. I help families look at how they can be financially empowered, and not simply dependent on government services.

KC: Why is financial planning and future care planning so daunting?
MS: I cry with people because of how afraid they are of this process, how scared they are for their children. People are afraid of what they don't understand. People often don't have a clear idea of what they want or how to do it. People don't want to look at their actual budget, because either they don't want to know how bad it is, or they're just afraid to know. But if you know, you can grow from there. I've been there with my own children, and I work with families to move away from being so afraid. Start the conversations. Tell your financial planner, "I need help."

KC: But I'm afraid of everything.
MS: I hear that. The biggest fear I hear is the fear of what will happen to a disabled child when the parents are gone. Families need to honestly answer these questions. Our culture has put it on people that they're terrible if they've gotten into debt or don't have an immediate plan for their children. This is wrong. Many people don't have the cash or the support system they'd like to have. There is **no shame** in wherever you are financially.

KC: Okay, so where do I even begin?
MS: Know what your needs are. What do you need now? In three years? In ten years? In more than ten years? Once you know this, you can plan your short-, mid-, and long-term needs. Include your dreams and goals. Look at your current budget and expenses, regardless of your credit score, debt, savings, etc. You need to know. Learn about ABLE accounts. If your child has an ABLE account set up, people can make tax-free contributions to the account that your child will be able to use for qualifying disability expenses, such as education, housing, transportation, legal fees, and health. Your financial planner can help you set up an ABLE account, often with as little as fifty dollars. You don't need a ton of money to get started.

KC: But you don't know my situation. It's just so stressful.
MS: In my own situation, with my own kids with disabilities, all that changed was knowledge. That was the light that changed everything: my stress, my sleep, everything. It's stressful enough taking care of disabled children. You can alleviate the money stress.

KC: Who gets my kids, including disabled adult children who are unable to care for themselves, when I die?

MS: That's for you to decide. Your special needs trust and your will include this information. For some, this is an easy decision. First choice, second choice, and a dozen people down the line just in case. For others, this is excruciating. Either way, you need to do it. If you do not designate someone to take custody of your children when you're gone, your affairs go to court, and a judge will appoint the person who will take custody of your child, generally the next willing family member. If you genuinely cannot designate a family member (and that's a reality for some), you can designate a trustee, such as a bank or an attorney's office, who is legally obligated to act in your best interest. Not ideal, but that's your alternative. If you can, avoid having a court sort out your affairs, especially your children. Get this in place as soon as possible.

KC: What if I did the work, but now I can't find the documents?
MS: Have a spot in your house with **all** of your paperwork, including printed copies of your ABLE account, special needs trust, life insurance, etc. Plus, have a printed list of how to contact your beneficiaries. You'll also want to have anything that sounds like an important legal document, such as power of attorney, conservatorship documentation, birth documents, and anything else that you think someone might need if you're not around.

KC: How much money do I need to save for my child's future?
MS: This depends on the child's needs. It's impossible to have one number that applies to everyone. You need to have enough to cover your child's expenses both now and into the future. The only way to know your number is to know your expenses now, and to project expenses into the future.

KC: What advice do you have for families new to figuring this out?
MS: You'll never regret saving too much. Government benefits can and will continue to change, and your personal financial plan is the only way to secure your future. Start by knowing where you are financially. There is no shame in wherever you are right now.

Conversations with Experts: Josh Fishkind

Josh Fishkind is the cofounder and COO of Hope Trust, a technology-based trust company dedicated to servicing disabled individuals and their families with a full range of financial planning and future care planning services.

KC: Do I really have to do this? My child is young, so I think I'll wait...
JF: Nobody likes doing estate planning. You don't know the day you're going to die. You need to make sure your child is protected on all fronts. It's nowhere near as bad to take care of this as people think it will be. Especially if you're working with people who have the right education and background in this. It's not on you to figure out everything by yourself.

KC: Should only rich people do this?
JF: No. This comes up a lot. Even families with really modest means need to consider how they're going to protect their loved ones. If more than $2,000 gets passed to your disabled child when you die, they'll get kicked off of their government benefits. They would get kicked off the benefits at the worst time: when you're not around. Sadly, I get these situations all the time. Don't be afraid to set up your plan. It is not cost prohibitive. The amount you will spend

varies based on the assets of the family and the complexity of the documentation based on your assets.

KC: I'm ready. I think. So, what now?
JF: Every plan has three components: the financial, the legal, the care. They are not distinct. They inform one another. All three of these should be done together. We start with the care planning. How much money is it going to take to enact this care plan for their lifetime? Talk to the financial advisor about how to get there, and the attorney about what legal structure is needed to manage that money in the long term.

KC: How many people do we need on the planning team?
JF: Ideal scenario: a financial advisor who understands your entire family's financial strategy, including your retirement plan, your life insurance strategies, your disabled child's financial needs, financial needs for other children; an estate planning attorney with special needs expertise; and someone to assess the long-term care needs for your loved ones. Others that can be helpful include an accountant and guardians who might be involved in your loved one's long-term care and support.

KC: What do I need to write into the care plan?
JF: What does a caregiver need to know that your child would not be able to communicate on their own? Make it as specific as possible. Include all daily routines and specifically activities of daily living. How does someone get dressed? How do they shower? Do they prepare their own breakfast? Are there dietary restrictions? Strengths and weaknesses. Likes and dislikes. Emotional resiliency. How do they do with money? All of these pieces may be instinctual for mom and dad but are a learned skill set for other care providers.

KC: Should the care plan also include how we envision our child's future?

JF: Yes. The child's future vision should drive the care plan. The best plans involve the person. That varies based on the individual. Let them know that a plan is being set up. Let them know a trust is being set up. Have your child participate, especially as they get older. I have disabled clients who are worried that their parents don't have a plan for their future. This is a concern they have as well. Can your child tell you who they would like to live with in the future? If they would like to take college classes? If they want to be out in the community more? Your child's goals should guide these conversations. Let them lead. These conversations are critical. "Nothing about us without us" starts with empowering your child to be a part of creating their future plan.

KC: How often should I update the care plan?

JF: Bring your team together every year. Review everything: financial, legal, care plans, trustees. Are the people you previously named still appropriate and able to perform these duties? If you're proactive with this, you'll sleep easy. You know if something happens, your care plan will be followed; there's a system. It's peace of mind.

KC: How can I prepare if there isn't someone to take care of my child in the future?

JF: Give your child a path. First, there's the financial piece. You can have a corporate trustee. It needs to be special needs specific; they need to understand Medicaid, Medicare, Social Security. There are trust companies out there. Guardianship can be harder. There are organizations in every state that will take on guardianship responsibilities. I suggest interviewing them during your lifetime to pick ones that you like. It is not a good plan to think the state will just appoint someone when you die. Meet with organizations and bring your child. Find the right fit. Participate in the process. Same thing with residential centers. I see aging parents whose disabled adult child lives with them, and the child is unable to care for themself independently. When the parents pass, the child loses their parents and their home at the same time. It is so much better for parents to look at housing options early, help their child transition, teach the group home staff about their child, tell them their child wants a Star Wars birthday cake every year—whatever makes your loved one happy. This is better than having a crisis when mom and dad are gone.

KC: How can parents best educate future guardians and trustees on the plans?
JF: You really need to educate them on government benefits, what you can pay for, how you get your medical supplies, what benefits someone is receiving and why. Getting it wrong causes a loss of government benefits. As to the care, there's nothing like firsthand experience. Show someone what your morning routine looks like. Teach them medical care routines, feeding processes, what are the tips and tricks for your specific loved one.

KC: I'm not sure where my child will be in terms of independence in the future, so I'm just going to wait and see. Cool?
JF: You will never hold your child back because you've done too much planning. Too often families avoid planning because they say, "I want to see how this turns out first" because there are so many potential outcomes for their child. There are flexible trusts and techniques. No one has ever come back to me and said, "I've saved too much money. I shouldn't have bought life insurance." If you plan correctly from the beginning, your plans can be extraordinarily flexible.

KC: What if my child isn't able to care for themself or to make legal decisions or manage their money or those sorts of things?

JF: Conservatorship or guardianship is an option to get another person legally designated to handle these affairs and legal decisions. It is a restrictive arrangement that isn't appropriate for everyone but can be necessary for those with extensive support needs.

KC: Is there another option? I'm scared of conservatorship because of Britney Spears.

JF: Your child may not need a guardian. In that case, supported decision-making can be put in place. You can work with your child, who's now an adult, to lay out frameworks—if a decision falls into this category, here's who you go to: your uncle is great with relationships, your cousin is great with money, etc. If your child is making decisions in conjunction with trusted decision-makers, this could be the best fit for them.

KC: If a child becomes disabled after the family already has a financial plan, does the family need to revisit their plan?

JF: The sooner you integrate your child's disability into the plan, the better. Families need to be aware that there are different age triggers. Disability before the age of twenty-two is a specific metric for certain government programs. Disability before age twenty-six is another. This will impact how certain government benefits play out in the future.

KC: Shhh, don't tell anyone, but I'm considering looking into a group home for my child when they become an adult.

JF: Families should consider all options. Residential programs can have long waitlists. Years. Start early. Involve your child. Where will your child be happiest? It's hard to think about, because you're a great parent. Is it better for your child to live with peers who share his disability? Is that what's good for him *and* for you? If you live to an old age, your child will be old too. Is it best for them to move out for the first time when they are well into their own adulthood? The programs will tell you specific criteria for what your loved one must be able to do for themselves in order to live there. If you're looking for things to focus on earlier, look at this. Does your child need to be able to do their own hygiene routine? Cook a meal? Your future plan can inform how you set goals from an early age.

KC: Once a family has this plan in place, if they move to another state, can it all fall apart?
JF: Unfortunately, yes. Many of these programs are administered by state offices. You need to apply for new state benefits, and know that not every state's benefits are the same. Before you move yourself or your loved one, get in touch with a government benefits expert and find out what programs are available, what happens to your Medicaid waiver money, can you still be paid as a caregiver? It can make a meaningful financial difference.

KC: What do families need to know that they're not thinking of?
JF: Talking to your family is a big one. Don't just assume a certain family member will step into future responsibilities. Is your chosen person truly ready to be your successor guardian? Show them what care means. Teach them about the feeding tube, the communication, emotional challenges, aggression, everything. It's rare that outside of the nuclear family people know what care really means. Be sure everyone knows about the special needs trust, be sure family members leave money to that trust, not to your child

directly. They can create a crisis if they don't know better. They could cause your child to lose government benefits if they don't have this information.

KC: What advice do you have for families as they begin their future care planning?
JF: This is long term. Work backward from your child's ideal future. Remove the shame. Talk about creating independence, agency, their best future plan. Empower yourself and your child.

Chapter 10: Everything No One Tells You About Inclusion in Your Community

Experts

Christel Seeberger
Sensory Friendly Solutions: www.sensoryfriendly.net
www.facebook.com/sensoryfriendly/
www.instagram.com/sensoryfriendly/
www.linkedin.com/company/sensory-friendly-solutions
twitter.com/friendlysensory
www.youtube.com/channel/UC9z7NWvtmO3dmEpdz74gj-A/featured

Paige Mazzoni
Canine Companions: www.canine.org

Katie Griffith
The Painted Turtle: www.thepaintedturtle.org
@thepaintedturtlecamp on Instagram
www.facebook.com/thepaintedturtlecamp

Gordon Hartman
inclusionstartshere.com

Morgan's Wonderland: morganswonderland.com
Gordon Hartman Family Foundation: www.gordonhartman.com

Parents

Donna Lee
www.stylingkindness.com
@stylingkindness on Instagram
www.linkedin.com/in/donna-lee-ma-nic-2a446345

Resources

Certified Autism Center
certifiedautismcenter.com

Disabled Parking
disabledparking.com

Inclusion Matters
inclusionmatters.org

Let Kids Play! (accessible playgrounds)
www.accessibleplayground.net

Project Angel Fares
projectangelfares.com

TSA Cares (Transportation Security Administration)
Passenger Support: www.tsa.gov/travel/passenger-support
Request TSA Cares Assistance: www.tsa.gov/contact-center/form/cares

The UD Project (universal design)
universaldesign.org

Conversations with Experts: Christel Seeberger

Christel Seeberger is the founder and CEO of Sensory Friendly Solutions.

KC: What should parents be thinking about when bringing disabled and/or sensory-sensitive kids out in the community?

CS: Feel empowered to make the decisions that your child needs. Set up yourself and your child for success with no apologies. Ask your children throughout the day: How do you feel? What do you need? Remember the basics: making sure your child has good sleep, isn't hungry or thirsty, has regular bathroom breaks. Build a toolbox, sometimes that's a literal toolbox of toys. Know what people and places work best for your child. It could be making a plan to leave early—and that's a healthy choice. Let go of the guilt, even if there is a cost of money or time or energy.

KC: What would you say to parents whose children have a hard time being out in public?

CS: Be as informed as possible about what the experience is going to be like. Many people can't just hop in the car and go. There are many barriers for some. Some places will have an accessibility coordinator that you can speak with in advance, or they will have accessibility information on their website. Look for that just right challenge for your child. Try new things. Sometimes it will work. Sometimes not. That's okay—and important. It comes back to finding out what sets up you and your child for success.

KC: I'm having trouble finding sensory-friendly experiences in my community…

CS: Find the people and environments that set you up for success. The difference can be the people; it can be the staff at the store. You might need to tell staff, "We need a different type of help." Think about what accommodations your family needs and communicate that—there will be others who would benefit from the same accommodations. Creating these spaces can be an unknown for businesses, so you might need to suggest steps they can take. Could your local grocery store have a regular sensory-supportive night that is open to all, where the music is turned off, the lights are lowered, there are fewer people, and a calmer experience? We can think about "turning down the noise" in public environments.

KC: What else should parents be building into their plans?
CS: Think about what you have the capacity to manage. As parents, we need to think about keeping ourselves regulated as well. Think about what we need so that we can be at our best and can be truly supportive. Involve your child in finding solutions. That helps them to understand themselves. Give children choice, empower them to understand themselves as sensory beings.

Conversations with Experts: Paige Mazzoni

Paige Mazzoni is the CEO of Canine Companions.

KC: What is the difference between a service dog and a pet?
PM: Service dogs are specifically trained to perform tasks for a disabled individual. Service dogs don't just provide comfort. They are there to perform specific tasks to mitigate the disability.

KC: How do I know if a service dog could benefit my child?
PM: The best thing you can do if you are considering a service dog for your child is to talk to service dog organizations to determine how your child could benefit. Service dogs can provide many types of services, including giving sensory pressure, fetching necessary objects, helping with exercises to strengthen muscles, and even providing a social bridge. Different organizations train dogs for different tasks so that the dog's skills can be tailored to the client's needs.

KC: A social bridge? What's that?

PM: A dog doesn't see the disability, they see their person. They form a bond, they become a partner to that child. They have a partner that's predictable, builds confidence, pulls people toward the child. When others, especially kids, see the dog, suddenly your kid is the cool kid with a cool dog. It enables interactions and friendships.

KC: My child isn't able to hold a leash or to give commands. Will that prevent them from getting matched with a service dog?

PM: The service dog can be placed with a two-person team, often a parent handler and their child, who are being matched with the service dog. The parent can facilitate and handle the dog in public, and the child isn't expected to manage the dog on their own. If you are part of a two-person team, both the adult and the child must be present for public access. In general, a service dog has public access; however, for places like school, religious organizations, and sterile hospital settings, you should get advance permission.

KC: Dogs sound like a lot of work. Are service dogs a lot of work?

PM: It's still a dog. They have extensive training, and you must keep up with that training. You have to take care of them. They become a part of your family, part of your daily routine.

KC: How do I know if a service dog organization is the right fit for my family?

PM: It's important to find an organization experienced with your child's disability. Ask how the organization works with the dogs and the clients. Make sure the organization is stable, and that they will be there for the lifetime of your partnership with the dog. Look for organizations that have high standards for quality and how the dogs are raised and trained. When that happens, you'll get a dog that is happy to be working and who is at their best as a working dog.

Conversations with Experts: Katie Griffith

Katie Griffith is the assistant camp director for The Painted Turtle.

KC: Your camp is fully accessible. What does that mean?
KG: Everything we offer at The Painted Turtle is designed so every camper has the opportunity to try it. The high ropes course is completely accessible for everyone. For children who use wheelchairs, they can literally zip line out of their chairs from the top of the course. We have no stairs and a zero-entry pool. Archery is accessible to all with adapted bows that operate with a flick of your finger to shoot an arrow. Everything was built to ensure everyone has access, and all the activities, spaces, and meals can be adjusted to fit the specific access needs.

KC: My kid has many support needs. I'm especially worried about their medical needs.
KG: Finding a camp that is considered a medical specialty camp is key. Look at the camp's medical team and see what conditions they serve and how much support they have on-site. At The Painted Turtle, we have a medical facility on-site staffed with a medical team that is well versed in all the medical conditions we serve. We also supplement each session with volunteer medical professionals who specialize in the particular condition we are serving. The Painted Turtle trains all our nonmedical staff members and counselors on the different illnesses to ensure we are fully prepared to serve every camper. In addition, we have a mental health team who provides behavioral support, which is vital in making the transition as easy

as possible. For some of these children this might be the first time they have ever spent a night away from home. Parents can call as often as they'd like to check in with us and see how their child is doing. It's our job to create the best experience for everyone.

KC: What can kids gain from a camp experience?
KG: Confidence is one of the biggest things. Kids conquer things at camp that they thought they never could do before—the ropes course, ride a horse, perform in the talent show. You see families drop off their kids, and everyone is nervous and anxious...then when the parents come to pick up their kids, they're a whole different child. Many campers don't know someone back home who has their shared experience. Finding people who can relate to what you are going through is one of the biggest gifts at camp.

KC: What would you tell parents who are considering camp for their kids?
KG: Camp is another way your kid can grow. This gives them such a sense of independence. They can do it. Camp provides confidence, independence, and a sense of fun—every kid needs that. Safety, fun, and connections are our goals, and we are able to achieve that. It's a beneficial activity that isn't just therapy. Camp is also a break for parents. We understand how important that is as well. It's exciting for the whole family when kids have this experience.

Conversations with Experts: Gordon Hartman

Gordon Hartman is the creator of Morgan's Inclusion Initiative, an organization focused on Ultra-Accessibility, which includes the world's first Ultra-Accessible theme park, Morgan's Wonderland, a sports complex, camp, Multi-Assistance Center, and more.

KC: Your organization focuses on creating Ultra-Accessible spaces. Why does that matter?

GH: All of my work is to try and put everyone on a more level playing field, to bring about more inclusion. The reason why I do what I do is because Morgan is one of the lucky ones. She has the doctors, the specialists, the team, and the support she needs. That's the exception to the rule. Morgan was the inspiration for our work, but it wasn't built *for* Morgan. It was built for everyone to access. We're taking "ADA-compliant" to a whole new level.

KC: You created the phrase Ultra-Accessible. Why does language matter when we're creating and talking about inclusion?

GH: Language does matter. It shapes our experience. In our organization, we don't "train" people, we *educate* people. When we're talking about Ultra-Accessible spaces, people can be clear on what that means. Individuals with disabilities are too often referred to as children. My daughter isn't a child, she is thirty years old. We need to look at and treat adults as adults. That's a mindset we work on a lot in respect to the community. Meet people where they are and treat them like the adults, and the *individuals*, that they are. There is no one experience of disability.

KC: Your organization includes Morgan's Wonderland theme park, Morgan's Wonderland Camp, Morgan's Wonderland Sports, Morgan's Inspiration Island splash park, and the Multi-Assistance Center at Morgan's Wonderland, The MAC. Why is it important to create such a variety of Ultra-Accessible spaces and activities?

GH: Everything we do joins people together. Ever since day one, we have been all about joining individuals who have disabilities with those who don't. At our Multi-Assistance Center, the individuals' families are involved. Anyone in the city can use our conference center. It's about everyone coming together. It's not about "those people," it's about *everyone*. With the Multi-Assistance Center, we are reaching more people to make sure they don't fall through the cracks. If they have doctor appointments they can't get to, we're making sure they have transportation. We want to build a fitness center where people can be working out alongside one another. We want to build an emergency room that is open to all, where the staff is specialized in treating individuals with disabilities. We've done many things and we're getting ready to do a lot more.

KC: That's amazing. When you say you're ready to do a lot more, what will that look like?

GH: We want to have a showroom for people all over the world to come to, where they can see what can be done. Does your community need to do this? We can show you how to do this. Does your community need that? We can show you how to do that. With the institute that we are building, organizations, companies, individuals, nonprofits can come here and understand how to become Ultra-Accessible, and fully inclusive. Our symbol is the butterfly, and when businesses become Ultra-Accessible, they can have that symbol posted so that people know that this an Ultra-Accessible space. We are creating a culture of more inclusion.

KC: Can other communities or spaces follow your lead in becoming Ultra-Accessible?

GH: They already are. Can anyone do what we're doing? Yes. We're not doing anything magical. We're just taking time out to ask how we can adjust and improve. Certain parts of Morgan's Wonderland are inspiring other parks, and they are adjusting according to what we have done. We're installing a thirteen-story zip line that allows someone in a wheelchair to go on it—they can have a breathing apparatus, a trach. We're engineering things that have never been built before. Everything can be done.

KC: What can all communities learn from Morgan's Wonderland's example?

GH: I want to make this a national and international movement, one that brings individuals with disabilities to the table. Right now, I'm working with a group in Philadelphia and a group in Saudi Arabia. Individuals with disabilities don't have a voice. We need to bring them to the table. I've met with political leaders, and this is a politically smart move. When politicians start to understand that, they jump on board. It's the right thing to do, *and* it gets them reelected. Fifteen percent of the population has a disability. And you're not just representing that fifteen percent. You're representing their families and extended families. This group is a multiplier. It reaches far into your community. We have both Democrats and Republicans coming together saying, "We need to do more." It's a matter of time and we will change the culture. Inclusion can be a catalyst for changing culture.

KC: What would you tell parents starting the journey of parenting a child with a disability?

GH: One of the benefits I had in my journey was that I was in the seminary for four years. We did apostolic work, meaning that we had to go and help someone for at least four hours a week. I worked with a lot of individuals with disabilities from a very young age. When Morgan was born, I had positive expectations of what her life would be like because of this experience. My wife had not had this experience, so she had to go through a grieving process. And that's okay. For us, the positives have far outweighed the negatives. Morgan has done so much for us. Morgan is my best friend. You have to be willing to be open to the thought that things aren't going to be exactly as you planned. At first this might hit you as a negative, but it *can be* a major positive. There is so much to look forward to.

KC: How can everyone start to make the world more inclusive, and ideally Ultra-Accessible?

GH: I often tell people to be curious. When you go somewhere, look around and ask: Is this Ultra-Accessible? Just think about it. Small things make a big difference. On our carousel, a wheelchair user can go up and down just like everyone else. It's a small detail, but to that person it's massive. Just look around and be curious.

Chapter 11: Everything No One Tells You About What This Looks Like for You as a Parent Caregiver

Experts

Amanda Griffith-Atkins

www.amandagriffithatkins.com

Jessica Patay

We Are Brave Together: www.wearebravetogether.org

jessicapatay.com

Brave Together podcast: www.wearebravetogether.org/podcast

Don Meyer

Sibling Support Project: siblingsupport.org

SibTeen: www.facebook.com/groups/SibTeen

Sib20: www.facebook.com/groups/118970768514797

SibNet: www.facebook.com/groups/SibNet

Briana Mills

www.brianamills.com

@BrianaMillsLMFT on Instagram and TikTok

Parents

Sarah Washington

www.makingmovesforme.com

www.facebook.com/sarah.washington.505?mibextid=LQQJ4d

Resources

American Psychiatric Association

www.psychiatry.org

American Psychological Association

www.apa.org

National Institute of Mental Health: Suicide Prevention

www.nimh.nih.gov/health/topics/suicide-prevention

Sibling Leadership Network

siblingleadership.org

Sibling Support Project, reference material for siblings

siblingsupport.org/publications/

Substance Abuse and Mental Health Services Administration

www.samhsa.gov/mental-health

Suicide Prevention Resource Center

sprc.org

Centers by states and territories: sprc.org/states/

Conversations with Experts: Amanda Griffith-Atkins

Amanda Griffith-Atkins is a marriage and family therapist, whose neurodivergent-affirming practice focuses on parent caregivers of disabled children.

KC: What emotions do you find parents of disabled children most commonly deal with?

AGA: Anything and everything. Most often grief, but that is shielded in so many other emotions. At its core, the grief is often wrapped up in sadness, anger, anxiety, depression. We aren't grieving that this child is ours. We are grieving experiences like calling 911 for seizures or finding a group home for your adult child who won't be able to live independently. It's not the experience you see on social media.

KC: Many of us feel ashamed to admit that we feel anything other than #blessed. What would say to people who don't feel they can admit their real feelings?

AGA: You need to find your people. Where can you be authentic with zero judgment? If you don't have those people in person, it's okay to connect with people online, find a therapist, journal. The more we are honest, the more it blows the myth out of the water that we aren't allowed to have feelings. With vulnerability comes healing. If you are able to be vulnerable about the realities of this, you give other parents permission to be honest about their realities. Saying this is hard doesn't take anything away from your love for your child.

KC: How do I know if I need therapy?

AGA: Take an honest inventory about how you're feeling: *On a daily basis am I feeling difficult emotions? Is it getting in the way of other parts of my life?* You might need therapy to work on processing one event, or to work on the big picture. Know your red flags of when you are starting to struggle. What are your signs of distress?

KC: How do I find the right therapist for me?

AGA: Talk to your friends. Talk to your insurance company. Interview therapists. Find the right fit. Ask directly if a therapist has experience working with parents of disabled children. If one therapist isn't a fit for you, ask them for a referral. As therapists, part of our job is to offer referrals. Give your therapist at least three sessions. If it doesn't feel right, it's okay to move on.

KC: I'm worried about how being a parent caregiver will impact my marriage.

AGA: Many things can get in the way of having a connected marriage. We are at risk because we have so many added demands. We have factors working against us that other families don't have: medical anxiety, financial stress, accessibility, advocating, and all of it. If you're not really working on your marriage, it will be impacted. Create connection from how you care for one another. Your relationship can too easily be centered on your child's needs. Focus on having a connected marriage. Both partners need to create space to listen. If you are the primary caregiver, your partner has to have an honest window into the caregiving life, the schedule, the therapies, the stresses, all the things. Be honest about how you're feeling. Talk about what this means for your family. Make that an ongoing conversation.

KC: How can I separate my own identity as an individual from my identity as a parent caregiver? Caring for my child is the most important thing in my life, and I'll be doing that forever. Do I get to be a person outside of that?

AGA: Parenting a disabled child often pigeonholes us into "that's my identity." So many parents, especially moms, start to lose themselves. Validate that. *Of course* you feel that way. Look at all you're handling day to day. Where are *you* in all of that? The person you used to be: What was important to you and is that still a part of you? That person has changed, but they're not gone. Honor the process of change. Reevaluate your expectations. Eliminate the expectation that we will reach mastery. This isn't something we reach the end of and then we start the next thing. This is not a destination to reach. Meet yourself with compassion along the way. You can be both a parent caregiver *and* your own person within that identity.

KC: But I'm exhausted. I feel like I'm giving and giving every day and I have nothing left.

AGA: That's called caregiver burnout. Signs of burnout are that you're not excited about the things you used to be, feeling hopeless, general exhaustion, feeling tapped out. There's lots of crossover with depression. This can be when you feel you're losing your identity, because you are constantly on call and always hypervigilant, like you're living for someone else. This is an alarm bell that you need to get some support. If you're feeling this way, I would encourage you to seek out therapy.

KC: People keep yammering about self-care, and even that sounds exhausting to me.

AGA: Think about what self-care looks like for you. Self-care can be doing the thing you don't want to do, like going to the dentist. You may not want to go, but take care of yourself like you'd take care of your child. Remind yourself that you want to have teeth forever. Think about where you feel good, where you feel alive. It could be sleeping, going for a walk, listening to music, checking out a book from the library—whatever brings you joy. You deserve to do the things that bring you joy.

KC: What do you think no one tells you about parenting a disabled child?

AGA: Don't jump to the wrong conclusions. You are not doomed. You're not going to lose yourself. You *can* still live a great life. There is joy. Life will look different than you ever imagined. You'll have more scars, but you can do it.

Conversations with Experts: Jessica Patay

Jessica Patay is the founder of We Are Brave Together, an organization focused on supporting mothers in the parent caregiving role through support groups, retreats, and resources.

KC: Your organization We Are Brave Together focuses on bringing together caregiving moms. Why is this so important?
JP: It can be highly stressful to have a child with a diagnosis or with unique support needs. Caregiving moms often experience isolation and compassion fatigue. We take that on by creating community, deep connection, and a sense of belonging. In our support groups and retreats, we bring together moms who get it, and it's transformative.

KC: What would you say to parents who feel isolated?
JP: Don't stay alone; don't avoid connecting. You can start with a group in person, or with an online community, whatever feels best for you personally. It is empowering to see the strength, the advocacy, and the incredible love that other moms have for their children. We can make each other brave by watching one another rise up.

KC: Do you hear common threads from many of the moms?
JP: Being overwhelmed but not knowing how to change that. Overwhelm feels terrible, but it's familiar, so it feels safer to stay stuck in it. Making change, trying to get help can feel scary. They can find they have trouble relating to friends who aren't in a similar situation. Moms isolate. Moms feel guilt for going on a walk or going out with a friend or taking time for things other than their child.

KC: So, mom guilt isn't just in my head?
JP: Mom guilt is real. When you have a child with a disability, the guilt can be exponential because the needs are exponential. You don't need to be a martyr mom, with no self-care and no breaks. Many moms think they need to do everything all the time for everybody, they think that to love is to give everything away until they're exhausted. That's a lie. It's unsustainable.

KC: What do you think no one tells you about being a parent caregiver?
JP: Acceptance doesn't equal giving up. The sooner we can accept that, the sooner we realize that our children are our greatest teachers, there's a piece that falls into place. Yes, I will advocate and push for progress, but I'll stop trying to fix; I'll ask what I can learn. There's such a shift and so much peace that comes with that. We can't discount our own personal journey to acceptance.

Conversations with Experts: Don Meyer

Don Meyer is the founder of the Sibling Support Project and the creator of Sibshops (workshops and peer support for young siblings of disabled children).

KC: Typically developing siblings are an important part of the family dynamic. How can we consciously support these children and honor their experience as a sibling?
DM: My work is to give siblings a forum in which they can talk about the good stuff and the not so good stuff with other people who get it, always in a very nonjudgmental way. I never tell kids

how they ought to feel about the situation they are in. Parents would be wise to acknowledge the ambivalence that siblings can have about one another, disabled or not. When you add a component of disability into the relationship, the highs are higher and the lows are lower. Some people say their sibling's disability is the reason their life is so screwed up. Some people say their sibling's disability taught them the meaning of love. Most often, it's somewhere in between. We need to honor the full range of experience. We need to validate siblings.

KC: What are Sibshops? Why does it matter for siblings to meet other siblings?

DM: Too often siblings don't have an opportunity to connect with other siblings. At Sibshops, we provide opportunities to connect in a relaxed, recreational environment that focuses on wellness. They are fun and lively, and kids look forward to coming back. The fun and recreation build the trust. Siblings feel validated when they meet one another and share experiences.

KC: What can parents do to encourage positive feelings about disability?

DM: The single strongest factor impacting a sibling's interpretation of their brother or sister's disability will be the parents' interpretation of the disability. If the parents view disability as a life-searing tragedy from which there is no escape, they should not be surprised if their typically developing kids view it this way. If the parents see the disability as a series of challenges that they need to meet with as much grace and humor as they can muster, then they have every reason to believe that their typically developing kids will feel this way as well.

KC: What emotions might my typically developing child be feeling?

DM: There can be a full range of emotions. Kids can have concerns, embarrassment, guilt, self-consciousness. They can feel guilty for arguing with their disabled sibling. Adults may even encourage them to feel guilty. Siblings may feel guilty for asserting their wish to be independent. There can be resentment when the family's world seems to revolve around their disabled sibling. There can be unrealistic expectations—many siblings grow up with a job description to take care of their sibling. Parents may fail to include typically developing kids in discussions of future planning, and not take into account all of their children's wishes. There can be pressure to achieve, to only bring home good news, to always be perfect. On the other hand, there are many opportunities. Maturity. Diplomacy. Responsibility. Advocacy. Humor. Insight into the human condition. Siblings may be better at standing up to bullies. Many siblings grow up to take on leadership roles, or to pursue care professions, such as doctors or teachers.

KC: Siblings can be the bridge to others, especially kids, who don't have experience with disability. How can we help our kids to feel good about these interactions?

DM: We need to realize that they won't necessarily want to be an advocate. The best thing families can do is to normalize the disability within the home. Teach kids about their sibling's disability. It empowers even young kids to talk about disability so that it's not stigmatized. Bring it up. Show them that it's nothing to be ashamed of. Build the conversation so that disability is just a normal part of life. Tell young kids that they didn't cause their sibling's disability and that they can't catch their sibling's disability.

For many little kids, they need to hear this. Every child's understanding of disability will evolve. Parents can provide a framework for conversation as kids age. Kids going into school will be asked—politely and not so politely—about their disabled sibling. They will be asked, "What's wrong with your sister?" Talk about that. Ask your kids what they say when people ask them that. They might have a great answer. They might not know how to answer, and this is your chance to give them something to say. Keep disability as an open topic.

KC: Should we involve siblings in making future care plans? Should we expect them to take on the caregiver role when they become an adult?

DM: We talk about self-determination with our disabled kids, but we can forget to also talk about it with our other kids. Self-determination applies to everyone. At the end of the day, it's the sibling's choice. We can increase the odds that they will choose to remain lovingly involved in the lives of their siblings. Do you want them to be involved because of a sense of guilt or resentment, or do you want this to be a loving choice that they have made? There is a range of ways to be involved. It looks different in each family.

KC: What can parents do to make sure their typically developing children feel equal in the family?

DM: Too many siblings feel invisible growing up. Let them know they are seen, they are heard, they are valued, they are validated. We ask siblings what parents have done to let them know they care. They remember the small things. They remember those things decades later. It's all about relationship maintenance with your children—with all of your children. Spend time with each child individually. Carve out the time. Give them permission to be less than perfect, and show them your unconditional love in that. The key is keeping communication as open as possible. Active listening is validation. And work to make sure your family doesn't have one person as the sun in your solar system. Find something that your family revolves around that reflects your family's values: soccer, basketball, your synagogue, your church, your community center. It can be anything. When it's not just focused on one human being, the family is about everyone and that benefits everyone.

Conclusion

Experts

Judy Heumann
judithheumann.com
The Heumann Perspective podcast: judithheumann.com/heumann-perspective
See the Conclusion for the full text of my conversation with Judy.

Parents

Kelley Coleman
www.kelleycoleman.com

Resources

Center for Parent Information and Resources
www.parentcenterhub.org

Disability Rights and Education Fund (DREDF)
dredf.org

ACKNOWLEDGMENTS

"You should write a book!" Great idea! And I couldn't have done it without a team of partners, supporters, mentors, and friends. I am endlessly thankful to...

My husband, Eric, you make everything possible and you make everything better. I am thrilled to be on this wild adventure together. My fearless son Sean, for your humor, empathy, creativity, and story notes. My in-love-with-life son Aaron, for the boundless joy that you infuse into everything. Even paperwork. I love the three of you more every single day.

The team at Hachette Go, for knowing from the start that this book will change lives. Dan Ambrosio, thank you for trusting me every step of the way and being an outstanding partner in the process. Nzinga Temu, thank you for jumping in and for always having answers to my many emails. Thank you to my publicity and marketing Jedi masters, Sharon Kunz and Ashley Kiedrowski, to Fred Francis, Monica Oluwek, and copyeditor Mike van Mantgem for making sure I appear to know what I'm doing, to Amanda Kain for your beautiful cover design, and the Hachette Go team working behind the scenes to make this book a reality.

My literary agent Laurel Symonds, for pivoting with me from fiction to nonfiction, beginning with your email that "this is both a surprise—and feels so obvious." Looking forward to many more surprises to come.

My brilliant writing group, for filling my life with inspiration, edits, and baked goods: Heather Dundas, James Sie, and Diana Wagman, without you this would just be a really long outline.

The mentors and fellow authors who guided me through the leap into publishing: David Ambroz, Kathy Hepinstall, Emily Ladau, Tiffany Yu and the Diversability Leadership Collective, and publicist extraordinaire Kelsey Butts.

The friends, family, and allies who keep me going: Shari Abercrombie, Jenna Boyd, Mindy Fishel, Rupinderpal Gill, Ben Gonzalez, Kaitlynn Hunker, Carri Kessler, Rachel Madel, Christina Mojica, Lisa Mosko Barros, Alyssa Parker VanOver, Beth Phillips, Jen Rarey, Kristin Rarey, Liz Rarey (hi Mom!), Allison Rawlings, Carolyn Sanchez, Hillary Seitz, Vikki Senna, Sloane Sevran, Kassia Shaw, Marini Hamilton Smith, Tarik Smith, Devorah Stark, Cecilia West, Cosette Zugale, and my online community members, who show up with grace, humility, candor, and humor. With extra high fives to Stephanie Bohn, Michelle Oricoli, and Sarah Washington for the races we've run (and won!) together, and for all the times you've dropped everything to take my calls.

The experts featured in this book, who taught me so much before we even spoke. Judy Heumann, I know you're looking over us all, hopefully satisfied that your work lives on.

The parents who contributed letters and stories, and all those who walk this path with me. Your stories and your children's stories will change, and perhaps even save, lives. We're in this together. Thank you for bringing me along on your journey.

And thank you to the enormous team of teachers, doctors, social workers, and supporters who have made our journey possible. Your wisdom and expertise have shaped not only this book but, even more so, our family and our future.

ABOUT THE AUTHOR

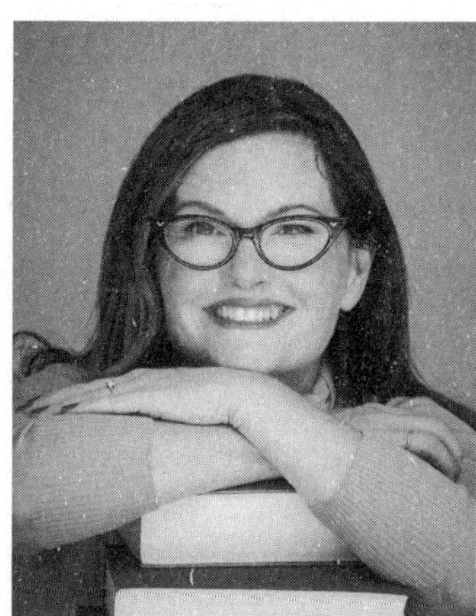

Photo credit: JTC Photography

Image description: Kelley smiles while leaning on a stack of books. Her arms are crossed and she wears a sweater and cat-eye glasses.

Kelley Coleman is a feature film development executive turned author and advocate for parent caregivers and individuals with disabilities. Her writing and advocacy draw upon more than a decade of experience accessing the supports necessary for children with disabilities to succeed, including her own. She serves on committees for Children's Hospital Los Angeles, the Los Angeles Unified School District, and Canine Companions. In her free time, she makes lists of things she would do if she had free time. Kelley lives in Los Angeles with her husband, two boys, her son's amazing service dog, and the thing that lurks beneath the bed.

www.kelleycoleman.com